# SELF-ADMINISTRATION OF DRUGS

## A Guide to Implementation

# SELF-ADMINISTRATION OF DRUGS

## A Guide to Implementation

CAROL BIRD RGN MA Clinical Practice Development Nurse,
John Radcliffe Hospital, Oxford
*and*
JANE HASSALL RGN DipN Ward Sister,
John Radcliffe Hospital, Oxford

*with 4 Contributors*

SCUTARI PRESS
London

© Scutari Press 1993

Published by Scutari Press, a division of Scutari Projects Ltd,
the publishing company of the Royal College of Nursing,
London.

First published 1993

**British Library Cataloguing in Publication Data**

Bird, Carol
  Self-administration of Drugs: Guide for
  Implementation
  I. Title    II. Hassall, Jane
  615
  ISBN 1-871364-82-5

Illustrations by Jean de Lemos

Typeset by Blackpool Typesetting Services Ltd, England
Printed and bound in Great Britain by Athenæum Press Ltd., Newcastle upon Tyne

# Contents

# Contributors

**Carol Bird** RGN, MA
Clinical Practice Development Nurse
John Radcliffe Hospital, Oxford

**Jane Hassall** RGN, DipN
Ward Sister
John Radcliffe Hospital, Oxford

**Neil Cottrell** BSc, MSc, MRPharmS
Specialist in Clinical Pharmacy
John Radcliffe Hospital, Oxford

**Chris Johns** RMN, RGN, CertEd, MN
Reader in Advanced Nursing Studies
Luton College of Higher Education

**Roderick Bird** LL.B
Solicitor

**Elizabeth Talbot** MA LL.B
Solicitor

# Introduction

Welcome to the book that has the potential to change the way you work. This book is about patients administering their own drugs while in hospital, but as the book unfolds, you will realise that the concept of self-administration is not just about patients taking their own drugs. The wider aspects include giving control back to the patients, empowering them so that they can make choices about their health and giving them the tools to ask questions.

This book will tell you all you need to know about:

- Setting up a self-administration scheme.
- The benefits of such a programme.
- The legal aspects and issues relating to accountability.
- The pharmacist's perspective.
- How self-administration improves compliance.
- How to convince other people that this is the way forward.

The editors of this book first implemented a self-administration programme in Oxford in 1987 using the framework described in this book. Since then we have been working alongside other health care professionals throughout the United Kingdom helping them to set up self-administration programmes in their own areas.

This framework has worked well for us, perhaps because it is comprehensive and easy to use. Self-administration is still going strong in Oxford and it has spread to many other wards in the hospital. Nurses and pharmacists from other hospitals in England have successfully set up self-administration programmes using our framework and more recently we have used the same methods to set up schemes in Australia.

This book should be of particular interest to nurses, doctors and pharmacists working in a hospital setting, and also to health care professionals working in the community, because the philosophy underpinning self-administration is applicable to all health care settings.

# 1

# The need for a change

I first became interested in the concept of patients administering their own drugs in hospital while I was working as a ward sister on a medical unit. The impetus for turning this interest into practice stemmed in the main from a feeling that a change in the system was urgently required due to what I perceived to be shortfalls in the conventional method of hospital drug administration.

At the start of every nurse's training, the importance of the nurse's role in drug administration is emphasised. The most important part of this role involves making sure that the right dose of the right drug is given to the right patient at the right time by the right route. I would ask, is this really the most important input a nurse can have in drug administration? What is the point of all this when we are going to discharge the patient home from hospital without the necessary information to get it right?

Safety, of course, is of paramount importance but does this method of drug deliverance ensure that patients will be safe when they go home? Surely there is a better way of administering drugs, one which would ensure that the patient not only receives the correct medication, but also understands why he or she is taking it, and how and when it should be administered. Clark-Mahoney (1984) applied the following adage to the way drugs were administered at the hospital where he worked:

> Take charge of administering a patient's medications, and he'll be compliant while he's in the hospital. Put him in charge, with supervision, and he's likely to stay compliant even when he goes home. (p. 41)

I would fully endorse this adage and it's probably the single most important reason to change your practice. I will now go on to describe the reasons for change in more depth.

Before embarking on a self-administration scheme for your patients it's important to explore your own beliefs about patient care, in other words your philosophy. We felt that patients should be as independent as possible, should participate in their own care, make decisions about their treatment in partnership with nursing and medical staff, and therefore be able to

1

make informed choices. Can you relate to these beliefs? Is this the sort of care that patients want? If the answer to both these questions is yes, then read on.

## THE CONVENTIONAL METHOD OF DRUG ADMINISTRATION

Does the conventional method of drug administration fit in with the beliefs listed above? Does it allow patients to participate in their care or make informed choices? I would answer no, it definitely does not.

The conventional system of drug administration is designed to protect the patient both from doctors' prescribing errors and from nurses' mistakes in administration. This system is primarily concerned with safety but does not make any provision for the patient to learn about and take responsibility for his or her own drugs. Although such a method is relatively safe, there are reasons why it falls short of the ideal. It is *only* relatively safe; this is borne out by the many drug errors made by nurses using a conventional drug administration programme. It does not incorporate a drug education programme for the patient nor does it encourage patient participation. The fact that patients do not engage in their own drug administration encourages dependence on the hospital staff and therefore may discourage patients from taking responsibility for other areas of their own health. This was the very antithesis of our beliefs about good practice in health care.

## HOW DO THESE SHORTCOMINGS AFFECT PATIENTS?

Through both my personal observations as a ward sister and discussions with community nurses, it appeared that non-compliance was frequently the end product of patients not receiving information about their drug regimens in hospital. Sometimes a patient would stop taking his medication because he felt better, or because he experienced a minor side-effect about which he had not been warned. Sometimes a patient would discontinue the drug when his hospital supply ran out, not realising that he was supposed to obtain a repeat prescription. Another patient might duplicate her medication by taking one frumil from her hospital supply and one frusemide from her existing drug supplies given by her GP. Other patients were unable to take their tablets owing to an inability to open the containers, perhaps because of decreased manual dexterity caused by arthritis or a stroke. The end product of these shortcomings was that patients were readmitted to hospital.

Let us now look at some of the literature which supports my personal observations. I noted that patients sometimes stopped taking their drugs because they experienced a minor side-effect. According to Blackwell (1973) the main reason patients stopped taking their drugs was because they developed a side-effect about which they had not been warned. The value of telling patients about potential side-effects is confirmed by the work of Wade and Bowling (1986) who note that patients may stop taking their medication because of a side-effect which may not be serious, or which may in fact be a symptom of another illness. Do you warn patients about the potential side-effects of the drugs that you give them? I certainly did not before using a self-administration scheme.

What about the statement that patients may stop taking their medication as soon as they are feeling better? Before carrying out my own research project, I was under the illusion that perhaps some people would stop taking a course of antibiotics maybe a couple of days before the course was due to end. In reality however, I found that some patients in my own study stopped taking drugs like digoxin or antihypertensives as soon as they were feeling better. Should this be such a surprise when we consider that many people are unaware of the purpose of the drugs they are taking?

Several authors have recorded incidents of patients discontinuing treatment, making errors or duplicating medication owing to lack of understanding. For example, Dunn (1987) studied the effect of hospital admission on the medication regimens of 52 elderly patients. Knowledge of drugs and the treatment regimen was not tested, but the effects of lack of knowledge were reported. Five out of the 52 patients had discontinued their own drugs. Three had used the hospital supplies and had not realised they were supposed to get more. One patient had stopped taking the drugs because he felt that he did not need them and another stopped the medications prescribed by the hospital because she preferred the drugs she had taken before admission. Fourteen patients had re-started drugs they had been on before admission to hospital because they felt it was the right thing to do.

Similar findings were noted by Hall (1981):

Patients discharged from hospital often continued to take the medication previously prescribed by the GP. This would sometimes cause duplication. The most common was taking one Lasix from one bottle and one Frusemide from another, not realising they were duplicating the same drug. (p. xiii)

Do you assess whether or not your patients can open medicine bottles or read labels? Is this really a significant problem for patients? Hatch and Tapley (1982) introduced a programme of drug self-administration, and they observed that some patients had great difficulty opening containers and many patients could not read the labels. Roberts (1978) also found that elderly patients experienced problems: patients with arthritic hands had difficulty when trying to grasp and manipulate small medicine bottles and many found the conventional-sized labels impossible to read. Again before introducing a self-administrating programme this is something I had never considered, and I certainly must have sent patients home with drug containers that they would not be able to open.

It appeared to me that all these shortcomings in the conventional drug administration system could be overcome by giving patients information, assessing for potential problems and allowing them to take their drugs under supervision.

## HOW MUCH DO PATIENTS KNOW ABOUT THEIR DRUGS?

Frequently patients appear to know very little about the drugs they are taking. Cartwright and Anderson (1981) studied a group of elderly people and found that one third did not know either the name or the purpose of the medication. Benson (1985) carried out a survey of 13 hospital in-patients. Patients were questioned to ascertain their drug knowledge. Eight patients thought they knew why they were taking the tablets, but not what they were called. The remaining five had no idea what they were taking or what it was for. MacGuire and colleagues (1987) investigated how much patients knew about their medications in preparation for implementing a programme of self-administration. They interviewed 23 patients aged over 65, only one of these patients knew the name, dose and effect of his drugs and even he did not know the frequency.

Ross (1989) studied the prescribed medication of elderly patients in an inner London GP's practice and was actually focusing on the discrepancies between patients and health professionals. As part of the study she assessed patients' knowledge of drug appearance, function, dose and frequency. The findings which emerged are shown in Table 1.1.

**Table 1.1**   Number of patient discrepancies of drug action,
from the work of Ross (1989)

| Patient knowledge | Number of disagreements |
|-------------------|-------------------------|
| Appearance        | 31 (12.4%)              |
| Function          | 71 (26.6%)              |
| Dose              | 47 (23.3%)              |
| Frequency         | 50 (20.8%)              |

n = 274 (number of drugs in the agreed regime)

Ross found that most discrepancies were about the patients' knowledge of the purpose of the drug and she gives a number of examples which include:

- Paracetamol 'for noises in the head'.
- Digoxin 'for the water'.
- Magnesium trisilicate 'don't know, but used to be for the bladder'.

Examples of disagreements on dose include:

- Patient reported taking neurophosphate – 'swig'.
   Agreed regime – 5 mls.
- Patient reported taking butobarbitone – two tablets.
   Agreed regime – one tablet.

Examples of disagreements on frequency include:

- Patient reported taking digoxin 'after a bad night's sleep'.
   Agreed regime – o.d.
- Patient reported taking thyroxine 'twice or three times a day under the tongue'.
   Agreed regime – o.d.
   (Ross, 1989: p. 133)

The fact that patients are often unaware of the name or purpose of their drugs suggests that they are not being given the information – or not being given the relevant knowledge in a format they can understand or can retain. Frequently this vital information may be given at the wrong time: for example, just as a patient is about to leave hospital or after consultation with the person's own doctor which many people may find stressful. The work of Higbee and colleagues (1982) illustrates this point. They surveyed patients who had been prescribed one medication at a clinic visit and asked them the name of the drug, the route of administration, the dose, when to take the drug and the duration of the course of treatment. Patients were able to recall correctly less than 50% of this information. I think that this highlights the importance of written information for patients, particularly to back up verbal information which is given when patients might have other things on their mind.

The reality that patients are frequently confused about their medications, because of the poor quality of the information they are given, has been noted by several researchers, and the resulting misunderstandings have been documented. MacGuire and colleagues (1987) give the example of a common misunderstanding occurring when patients are prescribed diuretics. These authors cite the case of a female patient who stopped taking her diuretics because they made her visit the toilet. She knew from experience the effect of the tablets but failed to appreciate the intention.

Wootton (1975) studied patients who were administering their drugs rectally. The findings revealed that nearly half the patients failed to remove the wrapper before inserting the suppositories.

## WHAT DO PATIENTS NEED TO KNOW ABOUT THEIR MEDICATION?

The Association of the British Pharmaceutical Industry (1987b) offers a list of recommendations concerning the quality and quantity of information about medications which should be given to patients. These recommendations include the following: written information should be given to reinforce the information given by the doctor and the pharmacist; the information should be brief and succinct, in a standardised layout, and aimed at a reading age of nine years; and an information leaflet should be included in the pack containing information such as how the medicine works, dosage instructions, method of administration, the times of administration, duration of therapy, administration precautions to be taken, and possible side-effects.

George (1987) reinforces these recommendations and states:

> The items covered should include the name of the medicine, when and how to take it, side-effects and what to do about them, precautions such as possible effects on driving, possible interactions with alcohol or other drugs, the purpose of treatment and how long to take it. (p. 1567)

## Do patients want more information about their drugs?

Hopefully I have put a good case to convince you, the professional, that patients need more information to understand the mechanics of their treatment regimen and this is obviously a prerequisite of safe drug taking, but do patients want to know more about their drugs? This is crucial because in order to create the right therapeutic environment and develop a partnership with your patient, it is important to give them what they want. Ley (1988) states that patient satisfaction is synonymous with the amount of information that a patient receives. This would suggest that giving your clients detailed information about their drugs will increase their level of satisfaction with their care.

Patients have also said that they would like more information about their medication. Cartwright and Anderson (1981) noted that the patients in their study felt that they did not know enough about their drugs. Ridout and colleagues (1986) carried out a survey of drug treatment using postal questionnaires; 740 adults in Southampton were sent the questionnaires, and 443 were returned completed. Two hundred and seventy five respondents (62%) felt that not enough was explained to them about medicines.

The work of Coutts (1979) confirms that patients do desire more information. In her study of gynaecology wards in Scotland, she found that patients wanted information on a wide range of matters. Oportunities for giving information were frequently missed by staff, low priority was given to patient education and staff were uncertain about whose responsibility it was to provide information.

### WHY DON'T PATIENTS RECEIVE ADEQUATE INFORMATION ABOUT MEDICATIONS?

It is apparent that health care professionals are in agreement on the sort of information which patients both need and desire to take their drugs safely. Why is it then that patients do not receive this essential information?

One of the reasons offered to explain why patients do not receive adequate information is that they don't ask questions. Meichenbaum and Turk (1987) suggest that patients are unable to ask questions because they 'do not know what they do not know'. Patients are not given the tools to ask questions and as a consequence are frightened of appearing ignorant.

George (1987) states that it is the joint responsibility of the doctor and the pharmacist to provide drug information, but notes that as both professions are busy they may forget! McEwen and colleagues (1983) suggest that education for improved medication may be a neglected aspect of care because it is not obviously 'medical'. They also note that it is not any specific professional's job to provide this information and each professional assumes that somebody else will do it, but in the end no one does it. This reminds me of a piece of graffiti which I saw written on a wall:

## AND THAT'S THE WAY IT IS!

This is a story about four people named Everybody, Somebody, Anybody and Nobody. There was an important job to be done and Everybody was sure that Somebody would do it. Anybody could have done it, but Nobody did it. Now Somebody got angry about that because it was Everybody's job, Everybody thought Anybody could do it, but Nobody realised that Everybody wouldn't do it. It ended up that Everybody blamed Somebody when Nobody did what Anybody could have done.

– Anon

In my own area, when using the conventional mode of drug administration, it was not automatic to give patients information about their medication. This was not because the nurses were lazy or because they did not possess the knowledge, but was due to the fact that this method of drug administration did not encourage it. Picture the scenario of a busy ward with only one or two trained nurses to carry out the drug administration for the whole ward. What is the main priority for this nurse – is it to get the drugs to the patient or is it to educate people about all aspects of their medication, check understanding, and assess for potential problems (e.g. difficulty in opening bottles, ability to remember to take the drug etc.)? Unfortunately, getting the drug to the patient had to be the priority, not education. This of course leads to dissatisfaction on the part of the nurse who feels that she or he should be sharing their knowledge with the patient, and for the patient who wants and needs the information which the nurse possesses.

There are of course other factors which influence whether or not health care professionals share this precious knowledge and these include the health professional wanting to maintain a position of control over both the patient and the situation, thus remaining in a position of power. This is supported by Stimpson and Webb (1975) who suggest that doctors tend to be selective with the information which they give to patients. They found that it was rare for doctors to name the drug but they would often make ambiguous remarks such as, 'I'll give you something for your nerves'.

This type of patronising manner was also noted by Isaacs (1979), who states:

> We tell them: 'never mind what it is – it's good for you, and doctor (or daddy) knows best'. But if patients don't know what they are being given, why they are being given it, and what good it is doing, they may see no good reason for going on taking it once they leave hospital. (p. 25)

This leads us on to look at what happens if patients are given insufficient information about their medication.

## WHAT EFFECT DOES THIS LACK OF INFORMATION HAVE ON PATIENTS?

The bottom line is that patients will not take the drug, or not take it as prescribed. The fact that non-compliance is a large problems has been documented by many researchers and will be discussed fully in the relevant chapter. Non-compliance is not the only negative outcome related to inadequate information, it does however appear to be the problem which is most frequently highlighted. I think that this is because it can be both measured and the cost estimated, which carries far more clout than other ill-effects which the patient may experience. What about the client's self-esteem? Does this suffer because of the fact they are not participating in their health care and are not taking control of decisions affecting their health? These issues will be teased out and analysed in the chapter related to the benefits of a self-administration programme.

## IN CONCLUSION

The literature reveals clearly defined guidelines for health care practioners relating to the information which should be given to patients to enable them to administer their drugs safely. It would also appear that many members of the health care profession, and researchers into the area of patient information, are in agreement as to what the necessary information should include. It is also apparent that the information which patients actually receive falls short of both the recommendations and what the patient desires.

To allow patients to self-administer their own drugs in hospital seemed to be the answer to many of the shortfalls of the conventional drug round. It allows patients to participate in their own care; it gives clients information; it encourages partnership between nurses and patients; and through giving patients all the information about their medication, including potential side-effects, it enables patients to make informed choices. These are the reasons why, in 1987, we felt the need for a change was sufficient to warrant the implementation of a programme of self-administration, and the following chapter will describe how.

# 2

# Implementation

There are a variety of ways of implementing a programme of self-administration. It is, however, important to use a framework of some description. Ideally, the decision to implement a programme should be a multidisciplinary decision, involving doctors, nurses and pharmacists. The commitment of the whole team is vital to the success of your programme.

The aim of this chapter is to give you a useful framework to work from when setting up your own self-administration programme. This is obviously not the only framework that you could use, but it has worked for me, twice, and has been used by many other wards in our hospital and by many others around the country. The chapter will explore some of the key areas, and hopefully offer some practical help on how to tackle potential problems.

## BACKGROUND RESEARCH

As with implementing any change it is essential to do your homework first, and in our case this took the form of a literature search. There are numerous articles written to date about self-administration and many will vary quite considerably in content and emphasis. The problem today can almost be where to start. What do I need to know before starting a programme?

Reading broadly around a topic is important. It certainly helped to give us a clearer insight into our own personal aims and objectives for a self-administration programme. It also enabled us to draw comparisons with other areas and to begin to visualise how a programme would work on our ward.

As well as reading articles, it may be beneficial for you to visit areas already using a self-administration programme. This is not because it is a visual thing, but it is certainly useful to talk to people who have been involved in implementing such a scheme. We were fortunate in Oxford to be able to visit Beeson Ward which was a nursing development unit at the Radcliffe Infirmary. Although this setting was quite different to our own acute area, we were able to begin to ask questions and to realise how we could adapt a programme to meet our own individual needs.

Exploring a new project can be time consuming and tedious. What is important is to set yourself a time scale and an outline of what you need to look at so that this stage doesn't go on indefinitely. It is all too easy to get off the beaten track and to review your results days later to find the correlated data is actually irrelevant to your needs. It is also possible to get overwhelmed with the amount of available literature, and you must be careful that it does not distract you from your intended goal! Our own review of the literature was quite limited to begin with and developed as our year of exploring self-administration went on. It is certainly useful to have a soul mate while you are conducting your research so that you have additional support and someone with whom to brainstorm ideas.

Initially our literature search was aimed primarily at exploring ways in which self-administration could be done. What did people actually mean by self-administration? We were totally preoccupied with safety and 'covering our own backs' – should we lock all drugs away, and if so, how? We spent many an hour poring over safety cabinet brochures and trying to find out from the UKCC and RCN, 'Where do we stand if something goes wrong?' We hope these questions will be answered as the chapters evolve.

### MOTIVATING STAFF

It is impossible to implement any new change without the full backing and support of the ward staff. So how do you motivate the staff? How do you encourage their willing participation in the programme?

From the outset, Carol and I felt it was essential that the project did not just belong to us, but to the whole team. We wanted to encourage their active participation from the very beginning. To do this, we obviously had to let all the staff know what we were hoping to do, but more importantly, to get them to realise why a change in the current method of drug administration might be necessary. The ideal place to reflect on one's own practice and to plan changes for the future is not necessarily within the hospital setting, and sometimes it is beneficial to get right away where there can be no interruptions. Although this is not always easy to organise, it should not be impossible, particularly if there is another ward with which you can exchange staff. It then becomes possible for them to cover you, and vice versa, for afternoons or days out as a team. This can provide an ideal opportunity to discuss major issues such as self-administration.

When we first told our staff about what we were hoping to do there were mixed reactions and a lot of uncertainty. They were certainly unsure about what the programme might mean and there was a great concern over individual involvement and what would happen if something went wrong. The discussions sparked off a lot of interest and it was useful that Carol and I had begun to review the literature so that we could answer the inevitable barrage of questions.

A majority of the staff at this time were new to the ward, which made us wonder if this was the best time to consider such a big change. On reflection this was a very good time since it meant as a new team they were starting together and working closely on a new project. It gave them a common and shared goal to work towards. Self-administration is not simply about letting patients look after and take their own drugs in hospital, it is also about attitudes to patient care, and encompasses general nursing ideology and beliefs. Self-administration provided us with the catalyst to start looking at other areas of our practice and was the impetus to review our ward philosophy. It was certainly relevant for us to look at our staff to see if any of them had previous knowledge or experience of self-administration.

Although, after discussion, everyone was in agreement about the overall inadequacies in our current drug administration system, there were notable concerns from the staff. There was a general feeling of how will this affect me personally? What happens if a patient overdoses, or if a patient forgets to take his tablets? Moreover, we had no comprehension about how this would fit into our already heavy work schedule. There was a reluctance to take on more pressure in a ward that was already stretched to full working capacity. I could certainly relate to these feelings. As a newly appointed senior staff nurse at the time, I also had reservations about the workload, how could I fit this into my already hectic work schedule? Would I be responsible for other members of staff? How would I be able to teach and supervise them?

The fact that we could work through a lot of these anxieties together was a tremendous bonus. We were able to work towards creating an atmosphere of mutual openness and support which encouraged us all to ask questions and to voice our concerns as we went along. As Carol and I continued to study the subject matter, our enthusiasm and motivation increased and with that so did the enthusiasm of the rest of the staff.

Perhaps one of the most difficult skills to master when implementing change is the ability to keep everyone informed as the project develops. This is important in order to maintain motivation and interest. Since implementation took us a year from day of idea to full implementation, keeping staff involved was of particular importance. Regular feedback meetings became a natural occurrence on the ward. These were frequently very brief and often took place during the shift handover, but it was enough to maintain interest. The staff were encouraged to go and review the literature themselves and to feed back their findings to their colleagues, and this helped them to develop a feeling of ownership towards the project.

Since implementing our programme, we have often been asked whether we ever considered it appropriate to introduce a drug education programme for our staff. The simple answer to this is 'No'. Although some staff had reservations about their actual drug knowledge, we felt it didn't warrant a formal educational programme. When I later implemented a self-administration programme on a haematology unit, I also chose not to introduce a formal teaching package. I felt that a formal drug programme would be off-putting to staff and would reduce their motivation for the subject. A formal teaching session went against the whole environment of openness and informality which I was trying to create. In reality, on both occasions, I found the latter approach satisfactory. There is no greater impetus for making staff improve their own knowledge than realising they have to chat to a patient about his or her drug regimen. Knowledge base can be increased by private study, utilising more senior staff and of course via your ward pharmacist.

So how suitable is this sort of environment for teaching students? At this time, students still did formal drug assessments so it was necessary to let the School of Nursing know what we were planning. We were totally confident, however, that we could offer the students a better education about medications by allowing them to participate in the self-administration programme, and we could assess student knowledge by listening to them telling a patient about their drugs. Since not all patients would be self-administering on the ward, this would also enable the student to experience both methods of drug administration. Students were always actively encouraged to participate in the self-administration programme under the supervision of a trained member of staff, and this helped them to feel more involved in the ward.

**TALKING TO PHARMACY**

One crucial factor in establishing a successful self-administration programme is the support and backing of your pharmacy department, for without this it is virtually impossible to implement a programme.

When we initially approached our pharamacy department, they were very enthusiastic. Certainly the idea, at this time, seemed very containable, and they were only too aware of the enormous problems of non-compliance. It is vital that the pharmacist is involved in helping to establish a programme from the very beginning since there are many key issues that need to be addressed and practical difficulties that need to be sorted out. What is crucial is that the nursing and pharmacy staff work closely as a team at all times. There must be thorough planning and a mutual understanding and respect for each other's pressures and constraints, but it is important not to lose sight of what you are both trying to achieve.

The programme has certainly helped working relationships with our ward pharmacist. When we first became interested in the concept of self-administration, there was no clinical pharmacy at Oxford, so our ward pharmacist would visit the ward once a day to check our ordering book and then leave. They had very little clinical input with staff, patients or doctors. Self-administration helped to create the right working environment to change this, because we needed to liaise very closely with our pharmacy department and our ward pharmacist from the onset to ensure the success of the project. We also needed their input in counselling patients about their drugs.

Carol and I were both concerned with the issue of safety and the storage of drugs for self-medicating patients. We felt that it might not be suitable for our patients to lock their medication and it was invaluable to be able to discuss our ideas and concerns with the pharmacy staff. It is vital that decisions about storage of medication are made by nurses, in conjunction with pharmacists, and that such decisions meet with medical approval. The multidisciplinary approach, advocated in Chapter 4, is of paramount importance.

Once our programme was implemented, it became apparent that the poor pharmacy staffing levels in Oxford would not permit the ward pharmacist to assess or counsel all patients self-administering, nor was this necessarily appropriate. What has been vital is to use them to troubleshoot particular problems that individual patients may be experiencing. We discussed at length the types of drug we were using on our unit, what would happen if a patient overdosed on these types of drug and what supply did pharmacy feel was appropriate to give our patients. Anxieties about the use of analgesics and supervising patients were also discussed.

The programme has certainly helped to open up the doors of communication between doctors, nurses and pharmacists. Our ward pharmacists are now heavily involved with teaching and educating both doctors and nurses on an informal basis and they have helped increase our awareness of potential common side-effects with medication and possible drug interactions. Through teaching the staff about the medication and by providing us with written information, they are helping to ensure that the patient receives consistent information.

Alterations have been made to the programme over the years, but what is important is that they have always been made jointly between pharmacy and nursing staff.

As interest in self-administration grew, and particularly after winning the Nursing Times Award, pharmacy were inundated with requests from other wards in the John Radcliffe to start a self-administration programme. Difficulties arose when wards made unrealistic demands of the pharmacy department, for example requesting to start a programme the next day, without even liaising with their ward pharmacist. The main difficulty for pharmacy is the additional dispensing time required to provide drugs for patients to self-administer. This is due to the fact that rather than just issuing a single ward supply of a drug, the tablets have to be dispensed in invidually labelled bottles, as with take-home prescriptions. The effect on pharmacy can be crippling if it is not done with thorough planning and, as mentioned above, it is important to recognise each other's constraints and to compromise accordingly.

We were able to identify quite early the key areas that needed changing and the constraints imposed by pharmacy were jointly agreed and have never caused a problem. More importantly, they have enabled the programme to run more smoothly. The constraints included:

- Not ordering at weekends or bank holidays when staffing numbers were low.
- Placing new orders for drugs for self-administering patients in the morning so that the pharmacists could plan their work-load.
- Having no more than three new patients starting self-medication on the same day.

We also try to limit the number of patients self-medicating at any one time to six, but this has never created a problem and pharmacy have always remained flexible and open to negotiation for different situations. For example, if a patient is ready to start self-administering and will be going home in three days' time, the pharmacy may agree to dispense his drugs even if he is our seventh patient, because they will not have to dispense any take-home prescription tablets.

The pharmacist's perspective will be covered in more detail in Chapter 7. My aim in this section was to draw your attention to all the positive ways your pharmacist's involvement can help you. I certainly wasn't aware, until I started working more closely with my pharmacist, of the valuable supply of ideas and various gadgets they had available for people with memory or dexterity problems.

There are tremendous 'spin-offs' for all patients on a unit which practises self-administration, not just self-administering patients. Our pharmacist is now seen as a valuable team member with a vital role to play in the clinical setting. It is important to work as a team, approach challenges and problems for your own individual areas together and adapt and compromise to meet each other's needs. The combined approach of pharmacy and nursing staff helps ensure the potential success of your programme and provides a constructive and progressive environment for your individual unit.

**HOW DO YOU GET THE SUPPORT OF YOUR MEDICAL STAFF?**

Approaching your medical team about self-administration can provide a stumbling block for many people who are trying to implement a programme. Do you need medical support, and if so, how should you go about getting it? The worst scenario is when medical staff simply say 'No' to an idea even without discussing the matter. Our doctors didn't actually say 'No – you can't do that', they just didn't seem at all interested in what we were trying to do or in our rationale for why a change was needed. They simply felt this was another 'little nursing study' and that we were tired of dragging the drug trolley around. They had no concept at this time of the wider benefits of a self-administration programme and thus could not appreciate our reasons for wanting to change, and were therefore reluctant to support us.

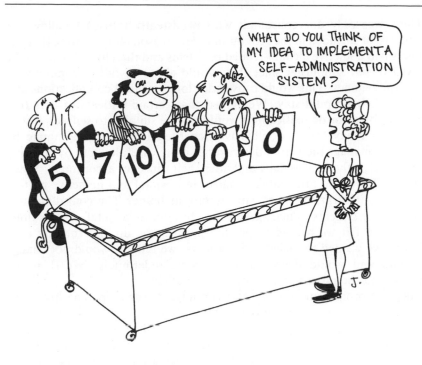

We were not necessarily looking for their 'permission' to start the programme, since storage and administration of drugs is the responsibility of the senior nurse and pharmacist in each ward (Duthie Report) but what we did want was their co-operation and support.

The aim of the programme was to provide a multidisciplinary approach with doctors, nurses and pharmacists all contributing to the patient's education. We were eager to move away from the scenario of doctors standing at the end of a patient's bed, discussing his treatment and progress, making alterations to his drug chart and then moving away without ever acknowledging the patient himself. We felt a self-administration programme would improve this situation since doctors would no longer be able to make alterations to the patient's drug regime without having to explain *what* and *why* to the patient.

We needed to let our medical team know what we were doing and initially we did this at a routine meeting. However, none of them appeared very interested in the idea so we decided to put it in writing. We sent a letter to all our consultants – we had four on our unit – and we also sent letters to two other consultants, one who was responsible for clinical practice within the hospital and another who had a particular interest in pharmacology. We worded the letter in such a way that, if they were happy for their patients to participate in the programme, then they needn't reply to the letter. Surprisingly, we had a mixed response to the letters, from no reply (which is what we expected) to enthusiasm and genuine offers of help.

There was only one consultant who persistently refused to allow her patients to be included in the programme. Her reasons for this were that her patients had addictive alcohol-related problems and therefore should not be allowed to self-administer since they would abuse or fail to comply with their drug regimes. This would cause additional medical complications and lengthen their hospital stay. We agreed that certain patients of hers (i.e. those admitted for detoxification) would not be suitable to self-adminster, but we felt many others would have benefited from the programme by learning to manage their strict diet regimes more carefully, and by enabling them to weigh themselves daily and alter their diuretics accordingly. When we were allowing so little patient control in hospital and no active participation, was it surprising it all goes wrong at home? The consultant was expecting her patients to manage at home but not in hospital. At this time, Carol and I felt we needed to get the programme up and running and, although we wanted to include her patients, we felt she would not change her mind and would delay the programme indefinitely. We therefore implemented the programme omitting her patients.

Once the programme was up and running, it was surprising how little interest the medical profession took. Many failed to realise what we were trying to do and one consultant actually approached me 18 months later saying 'It's here isn't it? . . .' having read about it in a local paper. We not only wanted their support, but also their participation, so their indifference at this time concerned us. But we realised Rome wasn't built in a day, and you don't change attitudes overnight!

It is important to have a multidisciplinary approach and the Royal College of Nursing certainly recommends that doctors should be actively involved in the programme. It is certainly beneficial to seek their advice and support about the self-administration protocol. Doctors needed more education and a greater understanding about what we were hoping to achieve and we certainly have more ammunition today to help convince them that this is the right way forward. Doctors need to realise the enormous benefits for their patients and also reassurance that we are not going to abandon patients once we have given them two weeks' supply of their medication, but will be providing assessment, support, and supervision on a continual basis.

Although different areas still have a problem getting medical staff to support them, it doesn't appear to be the enormous problem it has been in the past. Obviously, if they still remain unconvinced you can show them some relevant literature or discuss it further with support from your pharmacy or nursing management. They need to be reassured sometimes that this programme has been carefully worked out and planned with the patient's best interests being considered.

During a time of so much change in the Health Service and with innovations such as the Patient's Charter surely this is a time when all professionals need to reassess their own practice. Can we really, as individuals, continue the practice of giving no information to our patients?

## TALKING TO THE NURSING HIERARCHY

The structure of the nursing hierarchy has changed at Oxford since we first implemented self-administration. At that time the structure consisted of a ward sister, whose line manager was an Assistant Director of Nursing Services (ADNS) who was responsible for a group of wards, and then the Director of Nursing Services (DNS). The ADNS and the DNS were both unsure about how they could support and guide us when we first approached them. Discussions were hindered at this time by the fact that they really couldn't comprehend what we were hoping to achieve and why. The Director, of the time, could not commit himself to whether we should be allowed to pursue the project and felt the Assistant Director should make the decision for her clinical area. Unfortunately for us, our ADNS didn't feel she could support us with this project and she was particularly concerned with issues of accountability. We never did gain the support and backing of our ADNS nor our DNS. This lack of support was extremely disappointing. Everyone we had approached so far had anticipated problems, appeared sceptical and had put obstacles in our way, but we had rather naively assumed that our own nursing profession would be more supportive. Despite this setback, we remained firmly committed to the idea and felt so motivated and enthusiastic about the project ourselves that we decided to take a professional risk and continue with the project without their support.

We were fortunate in Oxford, however, to be able to seek the support and advice of Dr Sue Pembrey, who was District Clinical Practice Development Nurse. We approached Sue for some advice and were particularly anxious for some help to try and work things through with our nursing hierarchy. What was refreshing and so vital to us at this time was Sue's total support for the project. She felt it really was the only way forward.

At our request, Sue came to the John Radcliffe to talk to our senior managers with Carol and myself. It was important to have someone like Sue to show her support for the programme, but even this failed to convince our own nurse managers. Although Sue felt enthusiastic about the scheme, she could not take on all the responsibility herself. What she did advise us to do, however, was to begin to put something down on paper. This proved invaluable. At this time Carol and I had a lot of ideas and information about the project, but nothing in black and white. Sue recommended we went away and wrote a protocol. This sounded rather complicated to us initially – what did she expect? What should it include? We have been asked many times at our study days for a copy of this protocol. We do not give one, nor have we included a copy in this book for the very same reason. A protocol should be individual. It should be written by the ward team, including nurses, pharmacists and doctors and, if not written by everyone, it should be approved by all relevant personnel. Our protocol was very specific to our area, and it was essential to write since it helped us work through many of the issues. This proved important since it prepared us for when we were inevitably challenged about the project.

We kept the protocol as simple as possible. It consisted of a list of people involved in setting up the scheme – at that time, Carol, myself and our geriatric liaison sister. Our liaison sister had agreed to follow up all patients at home who had been self-medicating to enable us to get some feedback on the project. As a nursing sister working in the community, she was only too aware of the problems and difficulties people had with taking their medication once they got home.

We also included in the protocol our reasons for wanting an alternative to the conventional drug administration system, and our aims and objectives for the project. Following on from this we wrote in list form what we believed to be the main benefits of the scheme and alongside these what we saw to be the potential risks. We were aware that this sort of project is not black and white, and some sort of risk would remain. But we wanted to show that we had highlighted the particular risks for our own area and on this protocol we wrote briefly about how we would minimise these risks within the hospital setting. It demonstrated that we had thought through some of the issues relating to self-administration and the importance of this protocol is highlighted when you come to consider the legal aspects and issues of accountability. It is important that the protocol is agreed upon by the multidisciplinary team, doctors, nurses and pharmacists. Any recommendations must be agreed upon by all the staff working within the scheme and it is crucial that they adhere to this protocol.

Difficulties arise when people write one thing in their protocol but actually do something completely different in practice. Consequently, we paid particular attention to what was realistically possible for our clinical setting. We stated in our protocol that we planned to use an open system of storage for the patients' medication and gave the rationale behind this decision. What we particularly wanted to avoid was a situation where the protocol stated we locked drugs away, when in reality this was difficult to achieve and would therefore lead to a lapse in the protocol.

We identified the main risks, such as unintentional and intentional overdose, wandering 'Flossie' rummaging through lockers, theft and non-compliance. We felt all were manageable with some forethought and provision from the team because many of these potential problems would happen outside the hospital. So, surely, it would be better for any problems to be detected within a more controlled environment. It must be better for the patient to have the problem identified before discharge from hospital when there is a good chance it may be rectified. Who is there to detect a problem once a patient is discharged? Who is responsible once a patient does go home? Do we relinquish all responsibility when the patient is discharged? How can I be accountable if a person has been sent home with no information? Through writing the protocol we were encouraged to think carefully about self-administration issues, and to review our current practice and how 'safe' that was.

The benefits of the programme may be similar for each individual unit, but the risks will vary considerably depending on your speciality and age group. You need to identify potential risks in your own area and take appropriate action to minimise these risks for your particular client group. If everyone is in agreement with the protocol, it will not only help you to look at the wider issues of self-administration, but it will provide valuable guidelines to your ward and will not, therefore, be viewed as just another piece of paper.

We sent a copy of the protocol to our consultants, to the pharmacy department and to all involved members of the nursing hierarchy. Our original protocol was written solely by Carol and myself although, subsequently, when we have been setting up self-administration programmes, we have ensured they are written and approved by the whole multidisciplinary team. It was around the time of writing the protocol that Carol and I began to consider the issue of what documentation we felt was appropriate to use in this project. We were particularly concerned with the issue of assessment and information for patients and these documents will be discussed in the process and assessment chapters.

## TESTING THE WATER

Having researched the area, talked to members of the multidisciplinary team, written our protocol and documentation, we still remained hesitant about putting the scheme into practice. Despite all our work and enthusiasm for the programme, we had reservations about how it would work in practice. Can we really fit such a programme into our already chaotic day? Will the staff be able to cope? How will we be able to assess patients' suitability for the programme? There still seemed to be so many unanswered questions. We agreed that the only way to sort out these unanswered questions was by 'testing the water' and having a four week trial. In this way we could see the progamme in action and iron out any initial problems.

The purpose of the trial was to see if we could fit a self-administration scheme into our daily practice and to make any necessary adjustments to the programme. What was also crucial to us was that the trial should be successful and consequently we selected what appeared to be our easiest group of patients, those who had suffered a myocardial infarction. Here was a relatively young group of patients who often had a new diagnosis, little information and a new drug regimen and lifestyle to learn about. I became aware of the fact that this group of patients needed more information when I saw a 48 year old myocardial infarct patient practically crawling along the floor in front of the nurses' station when he thought no one was looking. He then pounced on the British National Formulary (BNF) which was lying on the bottom of the drugs trolley and scuttled back to his bed

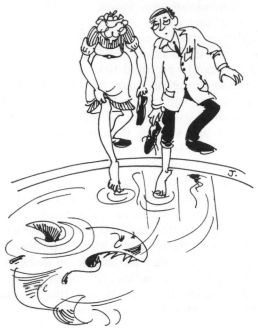

Testing the water

to pore over its contents. It suddenly occurred to me that far from being the advocate of education, nurses could instead actually act as a barrier to patients getting access to information. It saddened me to see this happening on my ward and even more so when I realised how unsuitable the information in the BNF really is for patients.

Jill, the geriatric liaison sister who was attached to the ward, automatically followed up any patients over 65 years of age when they were discharged from our unit. She also kindly agreed to follow up the patients who had self-administered their drugs, regardless of age, in order to provide feedback about the programme. We devised a very simple questionnaire for her to use during this follow-up period to ascertain whether we had improved patient knowledge and understanding in any way through self-administration. After four weeks, Jill's only comment was, 'Why are you only allowing patients who already know about their drugs to self-administer?' Of course this was not the case, particularly as the majority of the patients had a new illness (MI) and as a consequence, new drugs. This demonstrated to us that we had provided sufficient information for patients throughout the self-administration scheme, and this gave us enough positive feedback to continue on to full implementation. The four week trial also allowed us to see other positive aspects of the programme, most importantly that nurses did have the ability to assess patients for suitability to self-administer, and also that our documentation was suitable.

During this time only eight patients self-administered their drugs, but this was enough to allay most of our fears. We did not want to put pressure on to the staff, therefore starting small gave us plenty of scope to make adjustments and to support each other, and believe me, we needed this time as our anxiety levels were high! The most reassuring aspect of the whole trial was that it showed we could fit self-administration into our already busy day. More importantly, staff quickly realised how much they enjoyed and welcomed the opportunity to talk to patients about their drugs.

Regular feedback meetings continued throughout the four week trial and were conducted informally, usually at handover time. We would ask each other how things were going – were there any problems etc. It allowed us to sort out immediate difficulties very easily – for example, what about outliers? Should they self-administer? We decided no, since it was unfair to transfer them to another ward later on where the staff would take away this new-found control. However, as we adapted to the programme over the coming months, we would sometimes realise that an outlying patient had a glaring problem regarding his or her medication and, if we felt strongly that this patient should be taught and supervised within a self-administration programme, we would liaise with admissions and the doctors and request that the patient should not be moved to another ward.

Following the four week trial, we went on to full implementation. This went incredibly smoothly and I'm sure it was because we had been so

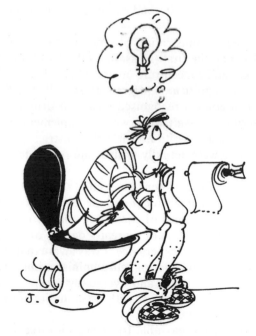

'It doesn't matter where you do the planning'

thorough in our planning and also working through the issues with other team members. No one wants to see a project fail, it is so disillusing. And once it has failed for whatever reason, it is so difficult to remotivate people and start again. Therefore, I cannot stress enough the importance of thorough planning, particularly when one starts looking at issues such as accountability and the legal aspects.

During the implementation phase, we found it beneficial to have regular feedback meetings with all personnel, i.e. pharmacists, doctors and nursing staff. This kept everyone informed about how the programme was going and enabled us to make adjustments together as the programme developed.

### SECOND TIME AROUND!

At the end of 1989 I commissioned and opened a new purpose-built haematology and bone marrow transplant unit at the John Radcliffe Hospital, Oxford. Immediately, I recognized the need to implement a self-administration programme on this unit. Here was a group of patients with serious life-threatening diseases, who needed to begin to understand their illness and future treatment. In doing this they would begin to regain some control over their lives. I knew from past experience that this could be encouraged through a self-administration programme since it would help the nurse and patient move more quickly into a relationship based on partnership. By entering into this partnership and by giving education, nurses help to promote trust and give their patients control and independence.

Implementing a self-administration programme the second time around was certainly easier than the first (Hassall, 1991). I was able to learn from my previous mistakes and concentrate on areas that I knew were important. Of course, there were significant differences as well, mainly in that self-administration had become a recognised means of drug administration in Oxford which it certainly wasn't when we first implemented it. Carol and I had, by this time, helped to write hospital and District guidelines for self-administration. (These were actually written approximately one year after implementation.)

The climate was certainly different the second time and it was refreshing not to have to battle with management and medical staff to gain support to do this. However, the principles of managing change remained the same and I was acutely aware this time of a greater danger of it becoming solely my project due to my previous experience. I was aware that the staff needed some time to explore the principles of self-administration for themselves to encourage them to feel involved, and eventually accept ownership of the project. Had it been just my project, with no commitment from the staff, undoubtedly it would have failed.

I was fortunate in that I was able to arrange a three week orientation period for the nursing staff prior to the unit opening. During this time,

I organised a self-administration study day for the staff which Carol and I facilitated. It was an excellent starting point and helped us to begin to look at the wider issues of a self-administration programme and what some of the possible benefits might be to our own patients. This prompted us to look at other areas of our nursing care, to challenge our ideology and beliefs. It helped lay the groundwork for us to begin to write our nursing philosophy. We were clearly able to identify that our patients had a right and a need for information and that this would be encouraged through a self-administration programme. It also highlighted the need to involve families in this extremely stressful period, and the fact that they too needed to be taught and educated and encouraged to participate, where possible, in the care of their relative.

Despite the fact that over 50% of the staff were new to the speciality, I decided against organising a formal drug education programme for them. I found that the self-administration provided an ideal vehicle for staff to learn about both drugs and conditions and, by promoting an open and relaxed environment, the staff felt at ease to question all members of the team and to use each other as a resource.

When implementing self-adminstration for the second time, I used the same framework that had worked for us before. We liaised with multi-disciplinary team members, rewrote the ward protocol using the same guidelines, and also used the same documentation. The framework has now been tested on a number of occasions both by myself and Carol, by other wards within the John Radcliffe, and by a number of hospitals throughout the United Kingdom. As a result, we now feel that we can safely say it works.

The main alteration I made to the framework the second time around was that I omitted a trial period. It seemed unnecessary since I knew it would work. I had previously tested all the practical difficulties and I felt I could guide the rest of the staff through it without having a trial group.

If you are thinking of implementing self-administration in your area, I cannot recommend too strongly the use of a small trial group prior to full implementation. There will always be teething problems with any change, despite all the preparations, and you have to be prepared to make adjustments as you go along in order to meet your own individual unit's requirements.

We had regular feedback meetings as before to enable us to iron out any difficulties. Any initial problems were soon picked up – for example, it was noticed that we were attaching rather expensive anti-emetic drugs to our drug reminder cards. This was stopped. It was also agreed that it was not good practice to attach chemotherapy drugs to these cards either, so this was also stopped.

Overall, the implementation went extremely smoothly and it was reassuring to find the framework worked just as well within a completely different setting.

**IN CONCLUSION**

Trying to implement a programme of self-administration may appear very daunting at the moment, particularly because there are so many plates to keep spinning simultaneously – maintaining motivation, getting the team's agreement, keeping good lines of communication open with everyone.

Sometimes while you are doing all these things it is very easy to feel swamped and disillusioned. Carol and I frequently asked ourselves, 'Why are we doing this?' It is important to keep a clear vision of what you are trying to achieve. Thorough planning and working through all the issues is an essential prerequisite prior to starting any self-administration programme. Once your programme is established and up and running, you will soon realise that self-administration is a dynamic process which requires continuous evaluation and adjustment.

By now you are realising, I hope, that self-administration is not simply about letting patients look after and take their own drugs in hospital. It is also about attitudes to patient care, about letting patients take control over their health and about health care professionals 'letting go' of their control.

With research showing that it improves patient compliance, drug knowledge and understanding about their condition, don't you feel it is important to at least explore the possibilities of implementing a self-administration programme in your own area?

# 3

# Patient assessment

This is an area which can cause concern and anxiety to many people wishing to implement a self-medication programme. The reason for this appears to be that it immediately highlights other areas of concern, such as personal accountability. People automatically link assessement with individual responsibility and assume that if anything were to go wrong in the future, then they as assessors would be held personally responsible.

At first glance, this seems a very logical conclusion and initially it was our own ward staff's greatest fear. We were constantly asked by staff, 'What will happen if something goes wrong?' and 'If I assess someone does that make me responsible?' To allay such fears and insecurities it is vital that staff have a clear understanding about the issues of assessment and accountability. They also need to know exactly *what* they are assessing, *who* should do the assessing and *when* and *how* this should be carried out.

## What are you assessing?

One of the most important issues to clarify in your own mind is what exactly it is that you are trying to assess. It is simply impossible to assess for everything, but how do you decide which are the key areas? It is also important to remember that no assessment provides a foolproof guarantee that nothing will go wrong.

Shortly after writing our protocol, we realised that some form of exclusion criteria for assessing patients' suitability to enter the programme was going to be necessary. We recognised that a framework for assessment was vital in order to ensure consistency, but it remained difficult to decide what were the key areas that we should be addressing. Carol and I both visited various wards and departments within Oxfordshire which were already using a self-medication scheme. Some of these areas had clear assessment criteria, others did not. The units we visited were care of the elderly

25

---

**PATIENT ASSESSMENT FORM FOR SELF-MEDICATION**

1.  Is the patient confused, or does he/she have a history       **YES/NO**
    of alcohol or drug abuse?
    (If yes, cannot self-medicate)

2.  Can he/she open bottles/foil packets?                        **YES/NO**

3.  Can he/she read the label?                                   **YES/NO**

4.  Have you explained what self-medication is to               **YES/NO**
    him/her?

5.  Have you explained:
    Which tablets/medicine he/she will be taking?               **YES/NO**
    The dosage?                                                 **YES/NO**
    Possible side-effects?                                      **YES/NO**

6.  After explanation, does he/she know when to take            **YES/NO**
    their drugs?
    (If, no, then strict supervision/instruction will be
    necessary)

7.  Have you given him/her a drug information card?             **YES/NO**


PATIENT ASSESSED BY: ................................................................

Date: ................................................................................

---

**Figure 3.1**   Patient Assessment Form

units which meant their criteria were different to our own requirements, although the principles of assessment remained the same. Our own assessment form, shown in Figure 3.1, has been adapted from Bradshaw (1987).

When we came to writing out our assessment form, we realised that it was important to keep it clear, simple and concise as nurses already have a phenomenal amount of paper work to complete. We felt that if we made the form too detailed or too time-consuming to complete, this would affect the nursing staff's commitment to the scheme. If staff were already anxious about carrying out assessments on patients, they would feel even less inclined to do so if the form appeared as complicated and ambiguous as a tax return form! We therefore tried to make it as straightforward and 'user friendly' as possible.

It is important that each unit should write its own assessment form using exclusion criteria which are relevant to meet that unit's specific needs. Our first question, for example, will not be appropriate to every ward. At this time, Carol and I were working on a gastroenterology and liver disease unit. We had a large number of patients with alcoholic liver disease related

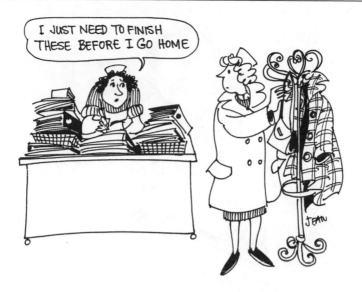

problems and we also had one consultant, mentioned in Chapter 2, who persistently refused to allow her patients to be included in the programme. Although we disagreed with her reasons, we had to comply at this time. Since 95% of this consultant's patients were known alcoholics, one exclusion criterion became possession of a history of drug or alcohol abuse.

Patients with liver disease problems, whatever their cause, can become encephalopathic and therefore confused. As this was a potential problem for our particular catchment of patients we wanted to highlight this risk to staff, and any patient who became encephalopathic would be withdrawn from the scheme.

Initially we felt any patient who was confused should not be included in the scheme but we have reviewed this since. We now feel it is more important to observe the reason for confusion (infection, dementia, encephalopathy etc.). It is relevant to know the cause since the confusion may be transient – if, for example, it is caused by a urinary tract infection requiring antibiotic treatment. The patient may not be suitable to self-medicate while confused from an infection but, following appropriate treatment, he or she would be reassessed.

As we have become more experienced with the programme, we now feel that our target group of patients needs to change. Originally (and wisely) we chose our 'easiest' and most *compos mentis* group of patients. However, we now actively target the more 'difficult' group since we realise that they will benefit from a closely supervised self-medication programme. It is important not to exclude patients who are normally slightly confused since these patients often have to manage their own medication once they go home, and surely it is better to start supervising them and to help them to establish a safe routine prior to discharge?

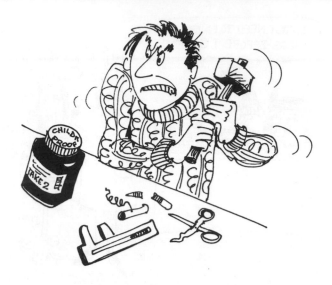

Some patients have difficulty opening their medicine bottles

Another key area that we felt was important to include in our assessment form was that of practical difficulties:

- Can the patient open the bottles?
- Can the patient read the labels?

According to Potter (1981) many patients may want to comply with their medication, but could experience difficulty in taking the drugs prescribed for them!

The fact that many patients have physical difficulties which make compliance more difficult has been confirmed by many researchers. Hatch and Tapley (1982) introduced a self-medication programme and observed that some patients had great difficulty not only with opening pill containers but also with reading the labels. Physical difficulties are not solely limited to the elderly as we at first presume; members of many different age groups find child-resistant bottle tops and small pharmacy computer labels difficult to deal with.

Originally, I had no idea what an enormous problem this was until I started working with a self-medication scheme. More importantly it was an area that I really didn't feel was my responsibility. Why should I check if people can open bottles? I automatically assumed everyone could or if they could not, then someone else would sort it out. It was not until I witnessed at first hand patients struggling with bottles and unable to read labels, that I realised that I had a responsibility to get this right – and, moreover, that it was essential to do so! We felt it was crucial, therefore, to include some check on physical capabilities for every patient.

If a patient is unable to read the computerised label this does not mean that he or she cannot self-medicate. Although a 'No' will be filled out on the assessment form, the nurse will then write next to this the action taken to meet the patient's needs. This can vary from providing larger print labels (which pharamacy are happy to do) or, sometimes, if the patient can't read, symbols can be used (e.g. moon and sun or colour coding). It obviously doesn't matter what the alteration is as long as it meets the patient's specific needs.

Until I started working with this programme, I was very ill informed about the enormous ideas and range of practical aids available from our pharmacy department for helping patients overcome physical difficulties. It became apparent that overcoming the patient's problem, when highlighted, was relatively easy. It was detecting the problem in the first place which proved to be difficult.

The rest of our assessment form acts as a checklist for staff. For example, has the nurse fully explained the self-medication programme?

Although we had managed to keep our assessment simple and concise, we were concerned as to how relevant it would be in helping our own staff feel more comfortable when assessing patients for the programme. We realised that what people appeared to want from an assessment form was a guarantee that nothing would go wrong and that the assessement itself could provide a 100% watertight guarantee. Is this ever realistic though? Can any assessment form provide such security? I fear not. Surely it is more important that the assessment covers areas that can be realistically assessed. It is important that staff are aware of what they are being asked to assess and that they feel such an assessment is feasible.

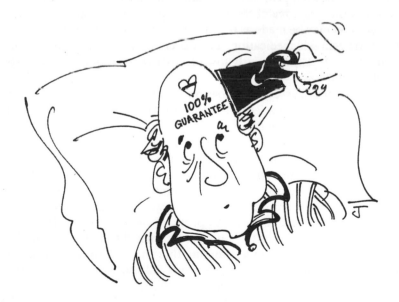

You may have noticed that we have not included anything on psychological aspects and many people ask should we not check that a patient isn't depressed or suicidal. Should we? Is this really a reasonable thing to ask your nursing team to do? I personally feel ill equipped to do a psychological assessment since I am not a psychiatrist. Can I really be expected to say whether a patient has a suicidal tendency? Can I honestly say if I know whether a patient is clinically depressed?

My own experience is that even psychiatrists find it difficult to answer such questions. On a previous ward where I was working, a psychiatrist was asked to see a patient because the nursing staff were worried about the patient's mental state. The psychiatrist saw the patient and wrote in the notes. 'This patient is not a high suicide risk'. Unfortunately, less than ten minutes after this visit the patient jumped out of a fifth-storey window.

It is important to look at this in its context. Do we, for example, assess patients' psychological well-being prior to giving them their take-home prescriptions? Does a doctor assess this prior to prescribing medication at a clinic visit? The answer is 'No'. This does not mean such areas are completely ignored. When I asked a GP whether he formally assesses a patient's psychological state prior to prescribing medication he answered, 'No, but I know my patient so I can generally sense if something is wrong'.

Is this not also the case with nursing staff who also work closely with their own patients? Don't nurses generally know the moment something is wrong and a patient becomes more withdrawn or anxious? In which case, if an alteration in a patient's psychological state was noted or a nurse was at all concerned, wouldn't he or she seek advice from other multidisciplinary team members prior to starting a patient on self-medication? In reality this is exactly what does happen. Any hesitation or concern on assessment is dicussed with other team members, including doctors and pharmacists, and a general decision may be made as to whether this is an appropriate time for this patient to begin self-medication. The patient may also be spoken to and asked if he or she feels particularly low or upset at the moment and, if so, can we help at all?

This sort of informal assessment goes on in every ward every day. Nurses work so closely with their patients that this sort of difficulty can and often will be detected. Although most nurses will be able to identify with this form of informal assessment and feel comfortable using it, this is very different to being asked to make a formal clinical assessment and to tick a box to say their patient is 'psychologically well' or 'will not attempt to commit suicide'.

People become very anxious about the limitations of assessments. What is important is you recognise the limitations, make a team agreement on what is appropriate and use that as your protocol and framework. Problems in assessment arise only if staff are unsure of what they are assessing for. They need guidance and an understanding that this is a ward assessment, agreed by the ward and which they can only fill out to the best of their ability using the framework provided.

Time to consider the limitations of assessment is important since it causes concern and considerable anxiety to many people who wish to implement a scheme.

**'How will I know if everything will be all right?'**

There is a fear of making a 'wrong' assessment and being blamed. Prior to starting the scheme both Carol and I were convinced that all patients coming into hospital and who were given their own medication would want to kill themselves! We felt the moment they had their hands on their own medication they would take an intentional overdose. Of course, in the cold light of day you realise that this is ridiculous paranoia. Self-medication offers a safe, supervised and educative programme for patients. Naturally, there are risks to any programme and what is important is to minimise these risks. You can help to do this by tailoring your assessment form to highlight potential problems for your own individual areas. Areas, for example, with children or a high population of confused elderly patients, or known suicidal patients need to devise their own criteria for assessment and decide what is appropriate.

So, on reflection, what exactly does this assessment form show you are assessing? It shows that you have considered the exclusion criteria for your own particular unit and that the patient meets these criteria (i.e. in our case, the patient is not a known alcoholic, does not have a history of drug or alcohol abuse and is not apparently confused). Our form also then shows that you have assessed some practical elements and are happy that the patient can open medication bottles and read the labels. It will also show when appropriate changes have needed to be made. The form also helps to provide evidence that someone has explained the programme to the patient, gone through his or her medication with the patient, given an information card and also checked that the patient has a reasonable level of understanding about his or her medication after the explanation.

This assessment form provides a framework and, by working within a framework, consistency will be achieved since each nurse will have to work through these key areas. It is important that the assessment form does tie in with the unit protocol as staff need to be aware of exactly what they are assessing patients for. For example, will patients be allowed to self-medicate any drugs or only a certain few?

When we originally started we were very concerned about patients self-administering on warfarin tablets, reducing steroid doses, analgesics and controlled drugs. We felt these were potential problem areas because doses could change on a daily basis and patients might not understand and therefore take the wrong dose with potentially disastrous consequences. Initially we didn't include any of the above-mentioned drugs in the scheme but, with experience and following discussions with our medical staff and pharmacist, we realised that it was appropriate to include these drugs on our unit, particularly since many patients went home on reducing doses of steroids, alternating doses of warfarin or high levels of analgesic medication. Changes were therefore made to our ward protocol and the staff were aware that following assessment, patients could also self-administer these drugs. Having worked through these issues my only advice is don't underestimate your patient!

As I have already mentioned, no assessment form is perfect, neither can you ensure that it will not fail. Many people have already devised assessment forms for their own areas, many others have also used or adapted ours. All I can say is that I have used this assessment format for many years in several different areas and have found it clear, easy to use and it has presented no problems for new staff using it for the first time. The fact that it has also been used and adapted by many hospitals throughout the United Kingdom and more recently in Australia, highlights to me the appropriateness of this format. Other forms we have seen over the years have included such things as mental test scores and assessing whether patients have an internal or external locus of control. Although this might be an interesting academic exercise, we do not feel this is necessarily an appropriate indicator as to whether or not patients can self-administer their drugs. Some people get so concerned about the issues of assessment that they forget all the benefits of the programme. You almost need to take a step back, think logically about what you hope to achieve and try it. No one can expect any more or any less, and, providing the assessment has been agreed with your multidisciplinary team and people follow the framework, you should feel relatively secure.

Assessment can always be adjusted and altered as you go along. Remember, we took a while to feel comfortable with this area and staff require constant support, guidance and feedback.

### WHEN IS THE RIGHT TIME TO ASSESS A PATIENT?

There is no particular right or wrong time to assess a patient for a self-administration programme. Some people feel concerned about whether it matters if it is shortly after the patient arrives on the ward or only 24 hours prior to discharge. There are in fact no set rules. Each patient will vary as to when will be the right time to start, but what is important is that it is the patient's decision.

I recently had a newly diagnosed leukaemia patient who was admitted to the ward for her first course of chemotherapy. During this time she was given detailed information about her diagnosis and treatment. The information we gave her also included talking about her medication. I filled in a drug information reminder card and showed her our documentation. Although she was very interested in the programme she felt it was not the right time for her to start since she still felt overwhelmed by the implications of her diagnosis. I have, however, had other patients who have been given the same diagnosis and have wanted to start the programme immediately since it helped them feel more involved with their care and treatment, and gave them a sense of regaining control over their own lives.

## Stopping and starting

Many patients coming into hospital for routine tests or surgery often remain on the same medication that they were taking at home. This usually means that the patient is already familiar with his drugs and, therefore, may be able to start on the self-administration programme immediately.

We have had many queries from nursing staff about what to do with patients who are self-administering but then need to have an operation. People tend to feel it would be disruptive to patients to stop and start on the programme and therefore would it be better not to include them? In reality, surgical patients are often ideal candidates for the programme. Many such patients come into hospital reasonably fit for a planned operation. They can be started on the programme prior to the operation and during this time you can also explain what will happen after the operation regarding their medication. Although there should be no blanket policy on self-medication for all surgical patients, it should be remembered that, for a period of time after the operation, patients may not feel up to taking their own tablets. This is often because they feel particularly nauseated from the anaesthetic, quite drowsy or in general discomfort. This needs to be explained beforehand. The severity of the operation, the speed of the patient's post-operative recovery or possible complications will dictate when it is appropriate for the patient to recommence the programme. In our experience, if this is explained to the patient before the operation, then problems do not arise and the patient is often just relieved to know what is happening. If a patient does self-administer prior to surgery, it often makes it easier afterwards when he or she may have to use a patient controlled analgesia pump (PCA). It is a natural progression then to go from the PCA pump to fully self-administering oral medication prior to discharge home.

The same principles for stopping and starting patients on a programme remain whatever the reason is for a break in the scheme. What is important is that it is always discussed with the patient first. There should be nothing secretive about stopping a patient self-administering even if your reason is that the patient appears a little confused. You should never resort to rifling through a patient's locker for medication bottles once the patient's back is turned. This is the quickest way to damage the trust that has been built up between you. Instead, talk to the patient, ask whether he or she is feeling a little confused, how is he or she managing with the medication and would it be more appropriate for the nurse to look after his or her drugs for the time being? Again, patients are often just relieved to know someone has taken an interest and I have never known a patient to be offended when I have had to ask them how they are coping with their medication.

It is important, when stopping and starting the same patient on the programme, that the patient is reassessed prior to recommencing self-administration. Even if the break has only been for a few hours, the fact that a break was needed for whatever reason also highlights the need to reassess the patient. The original assessment form can be used but it needs re-dating and re-signing.

The fact that a patient may be having problems on the scheme does not always mean that it is appropriate to stop them self-administering, sometimes closer supervision is all that is required. It is necessary to document any changes, however, and to explain new supervision plans in the nursing notes.

I haven't found a better or, for that matter, a 'worse' time to assess a patient for the programme. What matters is that the programme is flexible and customised to meet the needs of the individual patient. I have had many patients who have not self-administered until the day before discharge home; even this short time has shown itself to be beneficial.

I have, on occasions, kept patients in hospital for a day or two longer than planned because I have noticed a particular problem and felt more supervision and education was required. Even though we have a phenomenal bed crisis in Oxford and are always heavily pressurised to get patients home as soon as possible, a few extra days often stops the patient from bouncing back into hospital within a few hours!

### WHO SHOULD ASSESS PATIENTS?

Who exactly should do the assessment? Should it be a doctor, a nurse, a pharmacist or all three perhaps? When we started our self-administration scheme, whether doctors should or should not be involved in assessing patients simply was not an issue. This was purely due to their lack of commitment to the programme at this time and it certainly seemed very inappropriate for our own doctors to assess for something they had no interest in or understanding about.

If they had been heavily involved in setting up a programme, however, would it be appropriate for doctors to assess patients? Is this feasible? Certain considerations would have to include who in the medical team would do the assessing. For example, should it be a house officer, registrar or consultant? This immediately raises several practical considerations. If it should be a senior doctor, what is the likelihood of him or her actually having a close working relationship with the patient on a day-to-day basis? Will this senior doctor be around to provide ongoing assessment? If this isn't appropriate, is the house officer a suitable person? One potential problem is that house officers might be judged as too junior, or possibly on the ward for too short a period to provide any real consistency.

It certainly would not have been appropriate, on my own ward, for a doctor to assess the patients. This is purely because of the medical rota which means we have a fast turnover of junior doctors, and although their working relationships with patients are good, it is fair to say they do not work as closely with the patient as the nursing staff. This does not mean, however, that medical assessment is either wrong or inappropriate for other units, especially where medical input with patients is much higher and therefore ensures continuity on a day-to-day basis.

What about pharmacists? Should they be responsible for assessing patients? Again, there is no simple answer. It is important to look at the practicalities of whether a pharmacist will be able to get round and assess all the patients and how well he or she will know these patients. Even in Oxford, which is committed to clinical pharmacy, it has proved difficult for purely practical reasons for pharmacists to be the main assessors. It is also important to explore the relevance of pharmacists using their valuable time assessing patients, particularly on more specialist units where there is a high ratio of trained nursing staff.

In Oxford, many wards are using their nursing staff to do the assessment. From my own experience this has always worked extremely well. It has allowed our pharmacist more time to become involved with helping to teach and educate both staff and patients and to help 'troubleshoot' any particular problems we may be having. This doesn't mean that the pharmacist does not see the patient at all. Once a patient has been assessed for self-adminstration then our pharmacist will see the patient and chat to him or her about the medication and generally ascertain whether there are any outstanding problems. This provides a different perspective for the patient, and an excellent means of reinforcement.

### So why would a patient's nurse be suitable to assess patients?

Perhaps one of the most important reasons why the patient's nurse is a suitable assessor is because here is someone the patient knows and with whom he or she may already have established a good working relationship. Assessing patients for the programme should be carried out in a very informal and relaxed way. It should never be viewed as a 'test' that the patient has to pass. When we assess patients the form is often nowhere in sight and the patient certainly has no idea that he or she is being assessed for suitability. Instead we tend to incorporate it into their normal clinical nursing assessment.

Nurses have to ask patients awkward and personal questions about their health and lifestyle during the initial nursing assessment, so to ask patients about their medication at the same time would seem entirely appropriate. It often only requires very simple questioning to ascertain what the situation is, for example, 'What tablets are you currently taking?' 'Who normally gives you your tablets?' 'Do you know what they are for or why you are on them?' 'Do you normally have any problems with them?' It is possible to establish fairly quickly how much understanding patients have both about their medication and about their illness.

Many hospital wards now organise their work using team/primary nursing; with this system a named nurse is responsible for the total nursing care of each patient. Through organising the workload in this way, nurses and patients work much closer together and the relationship can become more like a working partnership where decisions, goals and objectives are set and worked towards together. This in itself provides an ideal forum to assess patients and to decide when is the right time for a patient to self-administer his or her drugs. Some patients will be ready to start immediately, others will require time and preparation. Due to their close working relationship, nurses can judge when is the right time for a patient to start and also how to stage the information. Meichenbaum and Turk (1987) noted the importance of pacing the nature and the form of education to the stage of the patient's illness. The patient's nurse will be able to judge more accurately the patient's frame of mind, many cannot cope with detailed information after they have first been admitted to hospital. At this time they are unlikely to be receptive to complex information about either their illness or the treatment. Later on, however, following the acute stage of illness, patients and their families are capable of giving their attention to the specifics of the illness and treatment regimes. The nurse can then customise the programme to meet the individual's requirements and can provide close support and supervision on a day-to-day basis.

It is important to realise that an assessment is not simply a 'one-off'. Patients require not only ongoing supervision but also continuous assessment. Problems do arise and it is important that everyone is aware of this. Many of our own staff originally worried that it would seem like a failure if a problem was detected and a patient was found not to be coping. Of course, nothing could be further from the truth since it is always better to detect any problem prior to a patient being discharged. I have often returned from days off to find one of my patients is no longer self-administering his or her drugs. A problem may have arisen, for example the patient may have become more acutely ill over the last couple of days and been seen not to be coping. I am never concerned or angry that someone else has changed my plans for a particular patient. On the contrary, I am always simply relieved that someone has been closely monitoring my patient in my absence.

This sort of scenario can cause tension and difficulties within some working teams. It is vital that the team work together and sort out problems and difficulties together when they occur.

Although I always felt it was appropriate for our own nursing team to be involved in assessing patients for suitability to the programme they were initially extremely anxious about this. It highlighted their own innermost fears regarding accountability and the age-old question of, 'What happens to me if something goes wrong?' It is essential that nurses feel supported. Our assessment criteria show that nurses have given patients information, assessed them for physical difficulties and checked that they have a

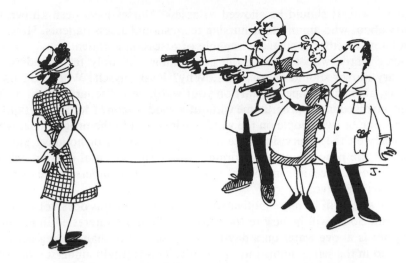

It is important to feel supported by your ward team!

reasonable level of understanding about their medication. Although the nurse signs the assessment form to show she has done this, does it mean she is personally responsible if something goes wrong?

Obviously she isn't signing the assessment form to say this patient is guaranteed to take his drugs as prescribed and that nothing will go wrong. Providing she is following the ward protocol and seen to be taking all due care, then the individual nurse and the ward as a whole will be in a 'safer' position regarding any possible litigation than if the nurse had not used any tool of assessment nor indeed taken obvious due care.

Certainly when we started our programme all the nursing team shared the same anxieties. They lacked supreme confidence in their own abilities and I remember distinctly the first patient we assessed was checked by five trained members of staff, 'Do you think he's OK? Would you agree to let him self-administer?' This acute anxiety syndrome lasted for a very short time. Once a staff member had assessed at least one person and nothing disastrous had happened within the first two hours, they relaxed and actually began to enjoy the programme. The nursing team soon realised they could do this; in fact it was well within their capabilities and much less of a major concern than many other decisions nurses are expected to make about their patients.

Nursing staff are routinely expected to assess patients and to prescribe and implement nursing care on a day-to-day basis. No one worries about this even though it may have more serious implications than a patient taking his or her own drugs in hospital under a well structured and supervised programme!

While working within a self-administration scheme over the years, I have always encouraged all trained members of staff to assess patients for the programme. Obviously it is the senior nurse's decision on the ward as to whom she feels should be allowed to assess. Nurses have been known to worry about who amongst the nursing team should assess patients. How *do* you know whether someone is capable of assessing a patient?

Some wards who are using the programme feel only team leaders or primary nurses should be assessors. Why? I ask myself. When you have willing, able and competent staff on your ward, why discourage them from being involved in the programme without a good reason? More importantly, if only one or two people on the ward are involved in the programme, who will carry on the supervision once they are on days off or holiday? Since I feel that the programme incorporates all our fundamental nursing beliefs and ideology, I feel it is important to encourage all members of the team to be actively involved.

Some staff will be more motivated than others, but this does not create a problem. Some will be new to the ward and be more interested in keeping their heads above water on a day-to-day basis rather than getting actively involved in the self-administration scheme. This is totally understandable – but to actively discourage staff from participating in the programme can be very demoralising and damaging to a team.

I have also actively encouraged student nurses to participate in the programme. I have always felt the original student drug assessment on wards was inadequate. Where was the skill, expertise or knowledge required in handing out drugs to patients, checking name bands and watching them swallow tablets? Since the final year students on our ward still had to do their 'drug assessment' it was necessary for us to liaise with the Oxford School of Nursing to discuss the feasibility of students doing their assessment on patients who were self-administering their drugs. This was not difficult to arrange since the School agreed that the student could be assessed by watching them assess a patient for the programme and by discussing the medication with the patient. What better way to ascertain students' understanding of the patient's medication and related illness than listening to them explaining it to a patient. Since not all the patients on our ward would be self-administering, it also meant that students would be exposed to two schools of practice and could subsequently draw their own conclusions as to the merits and disadvantages of each.

Involving student nurses in the self-administration programme helped them to become more closely involved in the ward and gave them an opportunity to create a closer working relationship with their patients.

Obviously each individual ward will have to decide what is appropriate for them regarding who should assess patients, the exclusion criteria to use and how ongoing assessment will be carried out.

There is only one hospital I am aware of that involves pharmacists, nurses and doctors in their assessment of patients. How this works in reality is not clear. If all three do assess the patients separately it must be extremely daunting for the patient, and if it is merely one person assessing but all three signing the documentation, is this either relevant or practical?

**IN CONCLUSION**

Although the assessment of patients remains a cause of concern for many people wishing to implement a self-administration programme, once it is up and running it in fact causes few difficulties and fits in as a natural part of the ward routine. What is vital, however, is that it has been properly thought out and that issues have been worked through with the staff involved prior to implementation.

There should be a multidisciplinary consensus about the framework for assessment and it should be made perfectly clear to those using it what the assessment form means, what you are trying to assess and who should do it. Initially staff need support and guidance with assessment but, once implemented, I have had very few problems either with the framework or with staff having difficulty using it.

The fact that Carol and I have used this assessment framework for a number of years in a variety of different settings and the fact that it has been used subsequently by many pharmacists and nurses around the country makes me feel I really can say it works. I hope it works as well for you!

# 4

# Self-administration – the process

This chapter gives a description of our process looking closely at what actually happens when a patient starts self-administering, the documentation that we use and particular problems you may encounter.

### PATIENT INFORMATION LEAFLET

Once patients have been assessed (see Chapter 3) as suitable to participate in the self-administration programme, they are given a Patient Information Leaflet (Figure 4.1) explaining what self-administration involves. A full explanation will also be given to each patient by his or her nurse, and the information leaflet can be used as a guide as to what areas must be covered in the explanation. This helps to ensure consistency. If the patient then wishes to participate in the programme he or she is asked to sign the information leaflet. The purpose of the signature is to provide written documentation that the patient has received an explanation about his or her drugs and the self-administration programme, and that he or she wishes to take part. What it does *not* mean is that all responsibility for drug administration has been transferred from the nurse to the patient.

The assessment form and the Patient Information Leaflet have been rewritten with the help of a solicitor. The decision to revise our documentation was made in response to the ward nurses', and indeed our own, increasing fears of personal accountability. These fears were mainly a result of the high profile self-administration was given after winning the Nursing Times Award in November 1988. Suddenly, we were inundated by nurses from other health districts who often asked very challenging questions about the programme, but also many others who wanted to use our framework and documentation. We therefore felt it was important to review our documentation, with particular regard to the issue of accountability.

The revised Patient Information Leaflet is a legal document which provides the nurse with greater protection because it demonstrates that information has been given to the patient, and it has the patient's signature. No system, however, is 'watertight'. Since at the time of this publication

### INFORMATION ABOUT SELF-MEDICATION

Self-medication is a programme used on this ward to help improve your knowledge about your medication. This is to help you to cope more easily with your tablets/medicines once you go home.

If you self-medicate in hospital it gives you the opportunity to take your own tablets under supervision. In order to do this your nurse will give you as much information, help and supervision as you need. Through this programme we aim to help you: understand the purpose of your drugs and how to take them safely; and to understand more about your condition and general health.

Before you take part in this programme you will have the opportunity to discuss with your nurse exactly what self-medication involves and what the possible benefits will be for you. Self-medication is not compulsory and you must not feel that you have to take part even if asked.

If you are asked, and agree to take part, then before starting a trained member of the nursing staff will:

1. Explain self-medication to you more fully.
2. Explain which tablets/medicines you will be taking.
3. Explain the dosage.
4. Explain any possible side-effects.
5. Give you a card showing your tablets and the correct dose, which you can keep and use as a reminder.

Your tablets/medicines will be given to you in bottles dispensed from our own hospital pharmacy. The bottles will have on them your name, the name of the medicine, and instructions on how often to take the tablets/medicine. You will be given a fourteen (14) day supply of tablets/medicine at a time.

PLEASE KEEP YOUR TABLETS/MEDICINE OUT OF SIGHT IN YOUR BEDSIDE LOCKER.

DO NOT EXCEED THE STATED DOSE.

IF YOU FORGET WHAT TABLETS/MEDICINES YOU HAVE TAKEN OR IF AT ANY TIME YOU HAVE ANY QUERIES THEN PLEASE TALK TO YOUR NURSE.

IF ANY VISITOR OR PATIENT TRIES TO TAKE YOUR TABLETS/MEDICINES PLEASE CALL A NURSE AT ONCE.

REMEMBER THAT IF NOT PROPERLY USED TABLETS/MEDICINES CAN BE DANGEROUS.

---

I HAVE READ THIS INFORMATION SHEET AND REQUEST THAT I TAKE PART IN THE SELF-MEDICATION PROGRAMME

Signed .................................................................................

Dated ..................................................................................

Patient name ........................................................................

Ward ...................................................................................

**Figure 4.1**  Patient Information Leaflet

no case, to date, has ever come to court regarding self-administration, it remains an untested law.

What is important, however, about our documentation is that it follows a protocol. It shows that you have assessed the patient to the best of your ability and offered explanation about the programme, also that the patient has requested to participate. Adhering to a protocol which has been agreed by the whole team reduces the likelihood of litigation.

A copy of this signed document is kept with the patient and a copy is put in the nursing notes.

### THE DRUG REMINDER CARD

It is vital that patients are given some form of written information about their drugs because it is often impossible for patients to retain all the verbal information they are given.

Research has clearly shown that drug reminder cards improve patient compliance. Ellis and colleagues (1979) carried out a trial in which patients were provided with written information about their drugs. Their findings demonstrated that the written information led to improved understanding and recall and improved both patient satisfaction and compliance. Hermann and colleagues (1978) also recommended that verbal counselling should be supplemented with written information.

The drug reminder card which we use for patients has been adapted over the years to meet our needs. Over a period of time we began to realise what information was useful to the patient and have added this to the card.

We decided the information should include:

- The name of the drug.
- How many tablets to take/dosage.
- When to take the drug/frequency.
- The purpose of the drug.
- Possible common side-effects.
- Special instructions.
- How long the course of drugs should be, continuous or short course.

It was reassuring later to find that the Association of the British Pharmaceutical Industry (1987b) offered a similar list of recommendations concerning the quality and the quantity of information about medications that should be given to patients. They recommended that information should include:

- Dosage instructions.
- Method of administration.
- The times of administration.
- Duration of therapy.
- Administration precautions to be taken.
- Possible side-effects.

To be effective and to aid compliance the card needs to be of value to the patient and therefore should be filled out using language that is familiar and meaningful to the patient. The card should be used as a reminder to the patient when to take the medication and to help establish a routine. This routine should definitely fit around the patient's day.

Meal times are often associated with taking tablets but not all patients eat three meals a day. Therefore writing 'Breakfast' 'Lunch' and 'Dinner' may not be suitable for certain patients. Also, not all patients have breakfast, lunch and dinner, but rather breakfast, dinner and tea. Some patients prefer to write specific routines they have at home on the card to act as a reminder – for example, 'After walking the dog' or 'After mid-morning coffee' etc. To establish a personalised and useful routine it is essential for the card to be filled out in conjunction with the patient.

It is the responsibility of both the nurse and pharmacist to help the patient establish a routine that is suitable for their medication regimen, and to write any special instructions for the individual medications on the card (such as take with food, after food or avoid alcohol etc.). We found that patients were frequently unaware of the medications which would make them feel drowsy and did not realise they should avoid driving or using machinery while taking a particular drug.

The actual name of a drug can also cause some confusion for patients since people often refer to the same drug by different names. The most common mistake is Lasix and frusemide. To help avoid confusion we always write both the name of the drug that the patient is familiar with, and also the generic name underneath. We also warn patients that the name, shape or colour of the tablet may change if their local chemist uses a different manufacturer. Therefore, we encourage the patient to take his reminder card with him when he obtains a repeat prescription so that the local pharmacist can alter the card if necessary. This is something our local pharmacists have been happy to do and it certainly helps to avoid confusion or mistakes being made.

A sample of the medication can also be stuck on to the card. Often patients find it beneficial to be able to visualise each tablet next to the instructions. They can immediately recognise the tablet and say, 'Oh yes, that's the one I take two of each evening'. I tend to ask patients if they would like a sample of the drug on the card to avoid appearing patronising, but I find a majority of the patients welcome this visual aid. Even patients who are only on one or two tablets and may have been taking the tablets for some time welcome the educational and visual reminder of the card.

Since tablets are stuck on to the card, we have written into our documentation and on to the card itself for patients to keep the card out of reach of children in order to meet safety regulations. We made a unit policy, however, that no particularly expensive drugs or chemotherapy preparations should be stuck on to the card. The reasons for this decision are obvious.

## GENERAL INFORMATION

If you experience any adverse reactions which you think may be caused by your drugs, KEEP TAKING THE TABLETS and inform your own doctor.

Obtain repeat prescriptions from your G.P. remember to telephone your doctor **before** your hospital prescription has run out.

Take **only** the tablets/mixtures which you have been given by the hospital. If you have any other tablets/mixtures at home, either return them to your doctor, take them to the chemist or flush them down the lavatory.

Please take this card with you to your doctor and chemist when you require more tablets.

Name ................

Address ................

................

................

G.P. ................

**Keep This Card Out of the Reach of Children**

| Tablets/Medicines | What Dose | Frequency | Special Instructions | Possible Side-effects (common ones) | Purpose | Continue or Short Course |
|---|---|---|---|---|---|---|
| | | | | | | |
| | | | | | | |

**Figure 4.2** Drug Reminder Card

Problems have occurred in the past when filling in the dosage to be taken. Previously, the staff would sometimes write one or two tablets instead of writing the actual dose in milligrams. The difficulty with this was highlighted by a patient who was taking 100 mg of spironolactone. During his stay in hospital the spironolactone was dispensed in 50 mg tablets and the nurse had filled in the chart – 'Take two tablets after breakfast'. When the patient was discharged from hospital a new prescription had to be dispensed because the patient had been with us for two weeks. His newly dispensed spironolactone was issued in 100 mg tablets. The reminder card was not re-checked prior to discharge and the patient continued to take two tablets instead of one. The error was corrected three days later at a routine clinic appointment but the incident highlighted two areas of concern. Firstly, the milligram dosage must *always* be filled out as well as the number of tablets to be taken. Secondly, all reminder charts must be re-checked routinely prior to discharge. The reassuring fact about the incident, however, was that it was the patient who questioned his dose of spironolactone at the clinic visit because he had noticed he was passing more urine. This incident also highlights the need constantly to review your programme and to make ongoing alterations when necessary to your practice and protocol.

We also write on the card whether the medication the patient is taking is a short or continuous course. Few patients are aware of this information on discharge and many patients will discontinue their medication as soon as their seven day take-home prescription runs out – being unaware of having to continue the medication or because they are unsure of where to get a repeat prescription. It is quite understandable that some patients only associate tablet taking with being in hospital and, therefore, once they are home and the tablets finished, they assume they are no longer needed. Unfortunately, the types of drug patients discontinue are not just short courses of antibiotics, but also other important medication such as antihypertensives, which are obviously vital to continue. The purpose of the medication is also filled out on the card. This is a vital component in improving compliance since what incentive does a patient have to continue taking a drug if he or she doesn't know what it is for?

The information on the back of the card was added after discussion with our doctors and the pharmacy department. The aim was to try and predict potential problems and thus minimise the likelihood of them occurring once the patient had returned home. We found that some patients took not only the medication given to them by the hospital, but also re-started medication that they already had at home. We therefore wrote only to take the hospital medication and to destroy or return to their GP any medication they already had at home.

Our own medical team were keen that patients didn't stop taking medication if they thought they were experiencing a potential side-effect, and therefore we wrote that patients should continue to take their drugs, but inform their doctor immediately.

The cards are made from cardboard for durability and can be folded into three, which allows them to be easily carried in a pocket or a handbag. We encourage patients to take the card to all doctors' appointments, to show them to their district nurse and also to their local chemist when obtaining a repeat prescription.

When we first started self-administration we never anticipated how well these cards would be used and it was a positive joy and delight to see them coming back weeks or months later all battered, much used and updated by various multidisciplinary team members.

### POTENTIAL SIDE-EFFECTS OF MEDICATION – SHOULD A PATIENT BE TOLD?

The question of whether or not to tell patients about the potential side-effects of their treatment is a controversial one and is frequently an issue where the medical profession disagree. Ascione and Raven (1975) revealed that 75% of physicians did not wish patients to be told about the potential side-effects of prescribed medication. This also appears to be the general feeling amongst many nurses as well. The overall fear seems to be that if patients are made aware or told about potential side-effects, they will not take their medication. Yet who should decide what patients should or should not be told? We strongly believe that side-effects should be included on the reminder card thus making the patients fully aware of the potential risks of their medication.

Although, as a profession, we are aware that in the past patients have not been involved enough in their care (and there is a desire, particularly within the nursing profession, to change this), we remain uncomfortable with the issue of telling patients side-effects. Is this because we should only tell patients nice things, 'This will make you feel better'? Or is it a dread that all patients will 'develop' the side-effect and stop taking a drug which the health professionals feel they need? Whatever happened to informed choice? Hasn't the patient a right to be given information and then allowed to make a choice?

The other area of confusion seems to be over 'what side-effects should we tell them?' I certainly don't think we should reel off the list in the British National Formulary. Obviously consensus amongst the multidisciplinary team is required to ensure that consistent information is given about side-effects. Realistically, the patient needs to be aware of *common* side-effects, which he may experience and cause him to stop taking his medication (e.g. headaches, dizziness, change in the colour of urine). The research actually points to the fact that patients are more likely to stop taking the medication if they are *not* told possible side-effects.

Bird (1989) clearly showed patients' anger at not being told about potential side-effects:

'I thought I was dying when the headache came on. I was very angry that I had not been told . . .'

If a patient does experience a side-effect such as headache or dizziness, it may not require a change of medication since it may only last a day or two and be expected. Other side-effects may just require a change in dose or switching to another medication. More problems are likely to occur if patients do not inform their doctor they are experiencing a side-effect because they may well just stop taking the medication that they think is causing the problems and, in doing so, are likely to stop the wrong medication. In order to achieve consistency of information for patients and to establish the 'common' side-effects of the drugs we were using on our unit, we liaised closely with our pharmacist and our medical staff and produced a written list.

We explored a core group of drugs we were using on the unit, highlighting approximately 20 main drugs. The pharmacist then wrote out a list of the common side-effects associated with these individual drugs, and this information was added to a sample reminder card drawn up by our ward pharmacist. The information on the sample card included normal dose, frequency, purpose, special instructions and side-effects of the drugs used in our unit and is referred to by all team members to ensure that patients receive consistent information. This information was later put into our ward computer, and both the medical and nursing teams find it a useful reminder. The information is updated by our ward pharmacist to ensure it remains accurate.

We are certainly moving into an era where patients expect to be given more information. The pharmaceutical industry have responded to this by proving written information leaflets with all their medication. In this age of increasing litigation, can we as health care professionals really afford not to be seen to be giving our patients information?

## STORAGE OF MEDICATION

This is an area which gave us considerable concern when first considering a self-administration scheme. How could we ensure that patients had free access to their medications and that the drugs were stored safely? We originally assumed we would have to lock all drugs away and therefore started looking at all the various locked cabinets and drawers that were available. Should we use a key, padlock or combination lock? Should we have one locked cabinet with individual patient drawers so that patients could come and ask for a key to get their drugs? Our concerns, once we started exploring the possibilities, were as follows.

Firstly, we were concerned that many of our patients would be excluded from the scheme simply because of manual dexterity problems which would prevent them from being able to open combination locks or use small keys. Secondly, as many other people will have found, to actually have drawers or lockers adapted would be very expensive. Thirdly, we felt many keys would be lost or taken home and what would happen then? Would we use a second key or have to change the lock again which would cause additional expense? The inconvenience this would cause the staff would also perhaps reduce their enthusiasm for the scheme and we were anxious to reduce the difficulties for our own staff at this time.

With a self-administration programme, we were trying to create a routine for patients that was as similar to their home situation as possible. We felt that by locking drugs away this might not create that environment since most people do not lock away medication at home and, to aid compliance, we had to create as few obstacles between patients and their drugs as possible. Simply making it more difficult for patients to access their drugs would possibly reduce patient compliance.

Finally, and perhaps most importantly, we were concerned about the interest that locked cupboards would generate amongst other patients, visitors or hospital staff. People would not necessarily be interested in the medication but in finding valuables. We had extensive discussions with our ward staff and our pharmacy department and, for the above reasons, decided to opt for an open system. In our ward protocol we highlighted our fears about the potential problems this could cause and wrote about how we would minimise these risks.

Our main preoccupation, naturally, was for safety. We emphasised how we would teach patients to be responsible for their medication, encourage them to keep it out of sight at all times in their lockers and to be particularly careful if children were visiting them. We felt this education about safe storage would not only help people while in hospital but would also be useful once they were at home. We also told patients to inform us if anyone tried to tamper with their lockers or medication, and we had these instructions added to our documentation.

Since we also had acute medical admissions from Casualty twice a week, we had our fair share of confused patients on the ward. We therefore highlighted in our protocol that confused or wandering patients would be kept away from self-medicating patients.

Our ward protocol stated that we used an open system and the rationale behind this. Although there is always some risk involved with using an open system, we felt that the benefits far outweighed the risks for our own unit and, as professionals, we recognised these risks and were prepared to take precautions and all due care to minimise them.

In all the years that we have been using this system, I can honestly say we have had no problems and I am aware of other units throughout the country who have also used an open system for many years and have also experienced no major problems. Obviously each individual unit has to look closely at its own situation and, together with the pharmacist, nursing staff and medical team, decide which system is most suited to its particular circumstances.

**Controlled drugs**

When we decided to introduce controlled drugs into our self-administration scheme, we decided on a slightly different storage method. It was agreed with our ward pharmacist and medical staff that these drugs would be kept locked in the patient's bedside locker. The drugs are ordered in the same way as the other controlled drugs but when they are delivered to the ward, they are first entered into the ward Controlled Drug Book, and are then signed out to the patient who signs that he or she has received them. In this way we have a record of how many controlled drugs are with a patient at any time. It was agreed with the pharmacist that when we started the programme a formal check should be made by the patient's nurse every three days to check that the patient has the correct number of tablets, that the patient isn't having any problems, and that no tablets have gone missing or been tampered with. Although this sounds quite formal, it is actually done very informally by the patient's nurse, and is a useful safeguard to alert the ward staff to any problems with patients mislaying or having any controlled medication stolen while self-administering on the unit.

**SUPERVISION**

People tend to assume that once patients are self-medicating they are then left to their own devices and no actual supervision takes place. This is not actually the case. Supervision at some level is always required, but what proved difficult when first establishing the programme was how this supervision should be carried out. Certainly when we started the scheme we were absolutely convinced that we wouldn't know if patients were taking their tablets or whether they were taking too many. We feared that unintentional errors would never be detected. Initially, we decided the only way to be sure that individuals were taking their medication was by performing a tablet count each day. This formal type of supervision lasted for two days! Here we were, on the one hand, showing that we trust our patients and are prepared to give them control through allowing them to self-administer, and then immediately taking it away with the other hand by performing tablet counts.

We soon realised a more informal approach to supervision was required. We discussed the issue with our ward pharmacist who agreed a tablet count seemed the wrong approach. It was decided by the ward team and the pharmacist that an informal check with the patient would be made once in every 24 hours by the patient's nurse. Due to the close working relationship the nursing staff have with their patients (i.e. team or primary nursing), it is not difficult for problems to be detected. Since nurses have good working relationships and since self-administration helps open doors to better communications between a patient and his or her nurse, problems are easier to detect. Often patients will admit openly if they aren't coping.

Some patients will ask for closer supervision or if a nurse feels that more supervision is required, he or she will discuss it with the patient and agree a suitable arrangement.

Often if a patient gets out his bottles of medication you can see at a glance whether the bottles are too full or too empty. Another way of detecting difficulties is through observation charts, i.e. the blood pressure is increasing despite starting antihypertensive drugs. We have had patients start self-medicating and subsequently a problem has been detected (e.g. they may be forgetting to take the drug). We view this as a bonus because it is far better to detect a problem while the patient is in hospital; it is too late after he or she has been discharged. Once a problem has been detected you can work together to find a solution. In all the years we have used the scheme, I can honestly say there has never been a problem with a patient that hasn't been detected by the patient's nurse.

The amount of supervision a patient requires should be decided on an individual basis. Carol and I have always tried to avoid any blanket policies to do with self-administration, since we feel each programme should be adaptable and be flexible enough to meet the needs of the individual patient. Some patients will be more than capable of self-administering immediately and will have minimal problems and will require minimal supervision. Others, you will soon realise, will need very close supervision and support and guidance until they are fully capable of self-administering their own drugs.

Initially it is always helpful to start with the easiest group of patients, but later on as you become familar with the programme you will feel more confident to tackle patients who appear to have more difficulties understanding anything about their drugs, or indeed about their illness.

Some people who have implemented a self-administration programme have gone down the road that all patients should be staged first (i.e. ask for their drugs first, have one day's supply etc. and build up slowly). Although I feel staging is a good thing, I do not feel it is appropriate – and it certainly wouldn't fit in with our nursing philosophy – for *all* patients to be staged. I have found staging appropriate for some patients but the amount of supervision has varied tremendously from patient to patient.

One patient I nursed couldn't read or write and was mentally subnormal. Not a good candidate to self-administer you may feel, but the reality was that he had had a massive myocardial infarct and he lived alone and would be responsible for taking his medication when he went home. It was impossible for his district nurse to give him his tablets every day even after we had simplified his regime down to twice a day. The only thing keeping this gentleman in hospital was his inability to take his own drugs safely. We therefore started him on a self-administration scheme with the involvement of the whole multidisciplinary team. Having simplified his tablets to morning and evening we had two large bottles sent from pharmacy with ordinary screw tops (not child-proof locks). On each bottle we drew a picture – one of the sun and one of the moon. We gradually built up slowly by asking the patient to recognise each bottle and to tell us when to use it. We eventually gave him one bottle containing one dose and left it with him to see if he took it. The whole staging and supervision took about a week and after this time the patient went home and, I'm delighted to say, self-administered his own medication quite safely without any difficulties at all.

This degree of staging was unusual for us. More often supervision requires working with patients who are not familiar with having to take their own drugs and find it difficult to establish a routine. Working closely with patients about their medication certainly helps them to build up confidence prior to going home. I feel many health workers underestimate how daunted patients feel about having to take their own medication.

It was agreed with the ward team that the drug prescription chart, which is kept at the end of the patient's bed with his other charts, would be checked at least once each day. This was a safeguard to ensure that if a new drug, dose, or alteration to any dose had been added by the doctor, it would be noticed. Although we aim for an ideal situation whereby the doctor would always inform the patient of any alterations, this does not always happen. If a doctor changes a drug and doesn't inform the patient or nurse, he or she could continue to take the wrong dose. In the ideal world, the doctor informs the patient, who can ask any questions he may have. The alteration is made to the prescription chart and the nurse/doctor or pharmacist will then alter the reminder card and if required, a fresh supply of tablets will be ordered for the patient.

We also came to an agreement with our ward team that in a 24 hour period the drug chart would be signed by a nurse to say he or she has checked with the patient that the patient is happy with the drug programme and is not having any difficulties.

### IN CONCLUSION

Initially, both Carol and I were concerned with the actual process of self-administration, and how well it would fit in with the day-to-day activities on the ward. In reality, it has created few problems and it soon became an integral part of our ward routine. The Patient Information Leaflet and the Drug Reminder Card have proved invaluable and both have been reviewed and altered over the years.

Obviously, each individual ward will have to decide on what documentation they wish to use, how to store medication for self-administering patients, and what format supervision should take. What does remain crucial is that all decisions have the agreement of the whole team and that, once a programme is up and running, it is regularly reviewed and altered when necessary.

# 5

# The benefits

This is obviously a vitally important chapter because it should demonstrate to you why patients administering their drugs in hospital is the right way forward. I also hope to demonstrate that the benefits of self-administration far outnumber the potential disadvantages and the difficulties of implementing and managing such a programme.

## ASSESSING THE BENEFITS

I am going to start this chapter by discussing each of the benefits that have been found by myself and other researchers in this field. I will try to illustrate where possible with patient quotes and case histories taken from my own experience, and from my own and other researchers' findings.

## Comfort

This is probably the most important benefit. Patients can take analgesics when they are in pain, night sedation when they want to sleep and tablets which need to be taken before, with, or after food, at the correct time. Generally people in hospital wait for the drug trolley before receiving medication and are reluctant to ask the very busy nurses for anything in between.

Many nurses seem to be frightened that patients will take too many pain killers either intentionally because their pain is inadequately controlled, or unintentionally due to the fact that they have forgotten when they last took any medication. The literature, however, suggests that this is unlikely. In fact several studies have shown that patients who have control over their analgesics are likely to take less than those who do not (Keeri Szanto 1979). Patients who have free access to their analgesics are going to feel more relaxed, they know that the drug is there when they need it and this should help keep their muscles relaxed. Picture the newly admitted patient, perhaps someone who has come in for pain control, sitting in a busy hospital ward surrounded by unfamiliar sights and sounds, who has had their analgesics

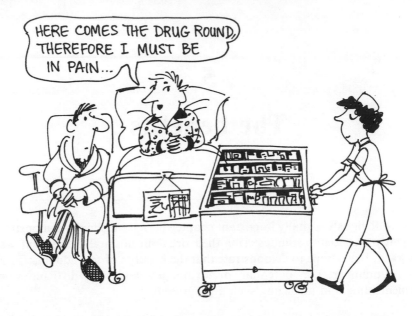

taken away when they entered the ward. How is this person going to be feeling? Are they going to feel relaxed and free from muscle tension? Or is it more likely that they are going to be panicking about where and when their next pain killers are coming from, and consequently will tense their muscles and actually worsen their pain. This cycle of tension and pain is represented diagrammatically by Gartside (1986) in Figure 5.1.

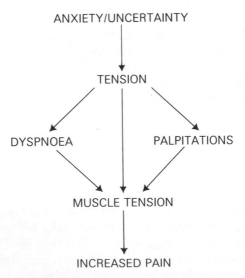

**Figure 5.1**   Effects of tension

I would like to illustrate the fact that drug self-administration improves comfort by describing a short case history.

### Brian

Brian is a 58 year old man who came to us jaundiced and in considerable pain and was diagnosed to be suffering from carcinoma of the pancreas with duodenal spread. The main aim of Brian's treatment was to control his symptoms.

Brian was prescribed:    MST 20 mg twice a day
Co-proxamol 2 tablets 6 hourly as required
Morphine Elixir for breakthrough pain as often
   as required
Lactulose
Docusate Sodium 200 mg at night
Temazepam at night

When Brian was first admitted and was undergoing investigations, his drugs were administered to him by the nursing staff. We found that we were not controlling the pain very well and after lengthy discussions with Brian I found that part of the reason was that he was not always getting his medication on time. He was finding this very frustrating but, because he was sensitive to the fact that the nurses were extremely busy, he had not liked to complain. Also, he had been informed by one nurse (who did not normally work on the unit) that he should not have medication prophylactically, but should wait until he actually experienced pain!

Brian was obviously an ideal person to administer his own drugs in hospital and he was assessed for suitability and given information about the programme. At first he sometimes forgot to take a drug (e.g. Co-proxamol which he was having for breakthrough pain) and so he devised his own record system by writing in his diary after he had taken a painkiller. He also devised his own pain chart from a standard one I had given him. Brian's system worked very well, after a few days he was able to chart the times of the day when he was getting breakthrough pain and instead of waiting for this pain to happen, he started taking analgesics prophylactically.

Because Brian had control over his drugs, this gave him some control over his pain and by educating him about the purpose of his drugs he was thus able to minimise his symptoms himself. Gradually, Brian was able to decide when the dosage of his analgesics needed to be increased and it was therefore possible to put the dose up before the pain was so bad that it would have required massive increases (with all the accompanying side-effects) to control his pain.

If the conventional system of drug administration is used patients may be discharged home from hospital without really knowing what breakthrough pain is, let alone how to control it. One of the reasons that this situation can occur is that nurses' knowledge about how to manage pain is inadequate.

Patient comfort is obviously a very important benefit, particularly in relation to pain. I hope that the example I have just given demonstrates that self-administration of medication would appear to maximise comfort and can even help to reduce the patient's pain.

## Independence

When people enter hospital they are stripped of their clothes and turned into patients, their individual preferences are frequently ignored, and they are often not party to the decisions which affect their health. All this results in a loss of independence compounded by the removal of their medication.

Allowing patients to administer their own drugs while in hospital helps to promote independence. If patients are less reliant on the hospital staff for their drugs it should follow that they may become more independent when it comes to other matters concerning their health. This is supported by Scriven (1987) who found that patients who had taken part in the self-medication programme which she instigated, felt that it gave them some control over what happened to them in hospital. Kallas (1984) noted that patients commented that self-administration helped them to feel independent and self-reliant.

Nurses and other health care workers are sometimes guilty of encouraging patients to be dependent on them, perhaps because they want to remain in a position of control and are thus keen to promote the unequal relationship of knowledgeable nurse and ignorant patient. I believe that we can no longer assume that patients are passive recipients of care but must actively encourage their participation and independence and self-administration of drugs in hospital is one method of doing this.

## Trust

Trusting patients has important psychological benefits for the individual patient. It also has benefits for the medical and nursing staff because if we demonstrate our trust for the person, they are more likely to believe in what we tell them and, perhaps more importantly, to act on this information.

I recently ran a seminar about establishing trust for a group of second year nursing degree students. When I asked them what they felt contributed to promoting trust, they replied that the most important feature was to be on an equal footing with the client. They felt that the best way to achieve this was by giving the patient information and allowing him or her to participate in decisions about his or her own health. Perhaps we have a lot to learn from these degree students whose new training is frequently criticised by a number of health workers.

Allowing patients to have control over their medication in hospital is a powerful way of demonstrating that you really do trust them. Many health professionals merely pay lip service to the concept of trust by telling individuals that, of course, we trust you to take your drugs, but then promptly removing all their medications from their control.

## Partnership/patient participation

I have already discussed that self-administration helps to promote trust and encourage independence. This, in turn, helps to change the patient/nurse relationship from one of passive patient/active nurse, to one of partnership. The patient and nurse become partners in care with potential gains for both, and this helps to promote a special sort of closeness which inevitably leads to an improved relationship between them. It is only when a nurse enters into a partnership with a patient that a therapeutic relationship can begin and the nurse is able to educate and motivate the client. This relationship may also help to raise the patient's self-esteem because it suggests equality rather than knowledgeable nurse/ignorant client. A 'spin-off' of this improved relationship is undoubtedly increased job satisfaction for the nurse: instead of merely administering drugs to patients the nurse is entering into a therapeutic relationship in which he or she is able to make the best use of skills – for example, by discussing the patient's illness and related drug therapy as opposed to just handing the patient his or her medication with little or no information.

Self-administration schemes also improve the relationship between the patient and the pharmacist. In the past on my own ward, the pharmacist would come on to the ward and just look at the order book and then disappear. Now, with self-administration, the pharmacist is a much more important member of the team. The nurses need their pharmacy colleague for information and to supply the drugs. Even more importantly, the pharmacist now talks to the patients – both to give them information and to help solve any problems.

We have also witnessed a change in the doctor/patient relationship. Before we used a self-administration programme, a group of doctors would often be seen around a patient's bed discussing the occupant's illness. They might then scrawl something on the drug chart and disappear. The patient was rarely included in these discussions and, as soon as the medical staff had gone, he or she would ask a nurse, 'What was that all about then?' This scenario no longer occurs because if the patient is responsible for his or her drugs, it is crucial that the doctor discusses any changes with the patient; otherwise the patient would not realise a change had been made. At first, doctors found this a little alarming. Now, however, they say that it improves their job satisfaction (particularly the junior doctors) because, instead of just carrying out the consultant's orders, they are discussing the implications with their patients. This is beneficial to both parties.

### Customised care

This follows on from the concept of partnership because, in order to ensure that care is customised, it is essential for the health care worker to enter into partnership with his or her client. An essential component of the self-administration programme described in this book is that it is customised for each individual. By that I mean that the amount of information required by each individual and the level of supervision required is tailor-made for every patient.

Some clients may already have an excellent knowledge of their drugs and have no problems remembering to take the medication. Such individuals would require little information (perhaps just discussion of common side-effects) and minimal supervision. Other clients might demonstrate poor understanding of the drug regimen and appear confused about when to take the drugs. They would require a specific programme of drug information, both written and verbal, plus close supervision. For example, at the start, patients may be asked to request their drugs when they think they are due. If this is successful then they may be given one day's supply of the medication and then slowly build up to a full supply when they are able.

Customising the self-administration scheme to suit each patient is a more effective way of helping clients to learn about their drugs. It enables the health care professional to build on existing knowledge through giving information at the right time for each individual patient.

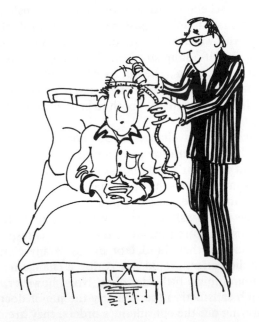

Self-administration is tailor made for each client

## Simplification

We frequently hear about the increasing problem of *polypharmacy*, particularly in the elderly who may have a number of different disease processes all requiring a different drug to treat. What can easily happen is that each condition is treated separately with a different medication and nobody actually reviews the diffuse drug regimen that the patient ends up taking. Wade and Finlayson (1983) reviewed the literature relating to polypharmacy and noted that many drugs taken by elderly people are either unnecessary or of doubtful value.

All researchers have noted that programmes of self-administration lead to simplified drug regimens. Nobody has offered an explanation as to why this might be. I think there is a very simple answer in that doctors actually witness how many different drugs the patient is taking when they are self-administering in hospital. Also of course the nurse is working very closely with the patient and so will perhaps be more aware that they are on vast amounts of drugs which could possibly be reduced. Bream (1985: p. 34) noted:

> By assessing a patient fully in self-medication we could help the medical staff to reduce the number of a patient's drugs to a realistic minimum.

As well as the nurse these newly educated patients will often suggest to the medical staff that the number of drugs they are taking could be reduced. A major benefit of simplification is improved patient compliance with their drug regimen. Stone (1979) reported that the rate of non-compliance rises from 15% when patients are asked to take one drug, to 35% if more than five drugs are prescribed.

## EDUCATION

Giving patients education about their medication is an integral part of a self-administration scheme because patients need information to enable them to take their drugs safely. Obviously the timing of the information giving is fairly crucial. There is little point in talking to someone about the finer points of their beta blockers when they are anxiously awaiting biopsy results to tell them whether or not they have cancer.

Meichenbaum and Turk (1987) suggest that, for patient education to be effective, the information should be customised for each individual depending on ability and phase of illness. A self-administration scheme is ideal for assessing the right time for a patient to be able to absorb the information and the nurse who is closely involved with that patient is the obvious person to note when the patient is ready.

My own research would certainly suggest that patients who had self-administered their own drugs had a much better knowledge of all aspects of their medication than patients in the control group who had not self-medicated (Bird, 1989). Bream (1985) also found that patients who had self-medicated in hospital had a considerably better knowledge of their drugs including purpose, names, dosage and relevant side-effects, than the control group. This is also confirmed by the work of Thompson and Ellenberg (1987).

The fact that a self-administration scheme improves patients' knowledge of their drugs is not really surprising because the programme incorporates continuous education which is both written and verbal, and it enables patients to practise drug administration under supervision. I also wondered, when conducting my own research (Bird, 1989), whether a self-administration programme would improve a patient's knowledge of his illness. My rationale for putting this forward as a hypothesis, was that through being given information about their drugs, patients were also given the tools to ask questions.

This hypothesis proved to be correct and patients who self-medicated were able to demonstrate a greater knowledge of their condition and the factors which may have contributed to their illness: 93% of the patients in the trial group who had self-medicated had a very good or a good knowledge of their illness compared to 43% of the control group. Only 7% of the trial group had a poor knowledge of their condition compared to 57% of those patients who had not self-administered their drugs.

The following patient quotes from my research (Bird, 1989) illustrate the difference in knowledge between the self-medication group and the control group. A trial group patient considered to have a very good knowledge gave the following account of his illness:

> I was admitted with chest pain which started as an ache in my throat and then became so severe that I actually collapsed. Apparently it is angina, severe angina, and in my case was caused by a high cholesterol level, causing a narrowing of the blood vessels to the heart. I know that I'll have to watch my diet now and they've given me a diet sheet.

This patient described his symptoms, gives the name of his illness and demonstrates that he understands the term angina. He also noted the cause of his illness and mentioned that diet control was a method of preventing recurrence.

Compare the above statement with the next comment from a patient in the control group who was admitted to hospital with a gastric ulcer and gave the following reasons for admission: 'After my last operation I was always getting wind and constipation so they sent me into hospital to find out why'. When questioned about the possible causes of his illness he replied, 'I've got no idea'.

I could fill a whole book with examples such as these, but hope that the two I have given are sufficient to illustrate my point; self-administration of drugs in hospital improves the knowledge a patient has of his illness. In what way does this knowledge benefit the patient? Well, it is back to the issue of informed choice and patient control. If a person does not have any insight into his or her illness and the subsequent effects on lifestyle, how can this person take control of his or her own health?

## ASSESSMENT

When a nurse administration system is used the patient's ability to open bottles and read labels is seldom assessed. The fact that many clients have difficulties in these areas has been noted by several researchers. Kendrick and Bayne (1982) noted that physical difficulties commonly hamper drug administration. They found that 13% of the elderly people in their study could not open flip-top pill containers, 53% had difficulty with palm turned caps, and almost two-thirds had difficulty with caps which required the lining up of two arrows.

A self-adminstration scheme allows the nurse to assess the patient's ability to open containers. In fact, this is part of the everyday supervision which patients receive. The scheme also enables the nurse to assess whether clients are able to take their drugs safely once discharged from hospital. For example, are they taking the drug as prescribed? Are they forgetting doses? Are they taking too many doses? Do they understand the purpose of the drug? Are they experiencing any side effects?

If a patient is experiencing any problems, these can often be rectified before discharge from hospital. Alternatively if the problems are insoluble then other ways of getting the medication to the patient can be explored, such as co-opting a relative or friend to supervise or administer the drugs, or perhaps involving community nurses. The end product of assessing patients' ability to self administer their drugs in hospital must result in improved compliance with drug taking. It must also reduce the risk of patients being discharged from hospital with bottles of tablets they are unable to open.

## Preventing readmission to hospital

Patients are commonly readmitted to hospital because they are unable to cope with their drug regimens at home. Youngren (1981) was aware that large numbers of patients were readmitted to hospital with drug related problems and termed this group 'revolving door patients'. The fact that this is a very real problem is confirmed by the work of Ausburn (1981) who assessed the reasons for admission to medical wards among a sample of 205 patients. The findings revealed that in 20% of cases the admission was probably, and in a further 5% was possibly, related to non-compliance with drug regimens.

Self-administration is likely to reduce this revolving door syndrome for a number of reasons. Firstly, the patient is given all the information about his or her drugs. Secondly the patient is allowed to look after his or her own medication. Thirdly, and most importantly, the patient practises taking the drug under supervision while still in hospital.

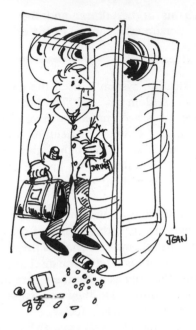

'Revolving door patient'

Compare the above situation with what normally happens in hospital. Patients have their drugs administered to them by nurses and often receive little or no information. They are not assessed to check whether they can open bottles or read labels. They are given no opportunity to practise drug administration under supervision. If there is a problem, therefore, it will not be detected. With this in mind it is hardly surprising that these clients bounce back into hospital with drug related problems.

Self-administration schemes may extend the time some patients spend in hospital because if they do experience a problem, then obviously they cannot be discharged home until it has been resolved. The self-administration programme must, however, be more cost effective, and more satisfactory for the patient, than readmission to hospital with all the emotional and practical problems incumbent upon this.

### PATIENT CONTROL

Giving patients control of their drugs is a crucial part of the self-administration scheme and I strongly believe that giving clients this control may help them to retain, or in some cases regain, control over their health. The main reason that a self-administration programme enables patients to regain control over their health, is that it changes the ethos of the ward from one of doing to people, to one of educating and motivating clients to make informed choices about their health. This is empowerment.

I have already discussed how self-administration helps the nurse to enter into a partnership with the client through trust and information giving. Once this relationship has been entered into, it is actually possible to help motivate patients to accept the control of and responsibility for their drugs and ultimately their health.

Establishing the nurse/patient relationship is a crucial part of enabling clients to take control because it is only when a partnership has been formed that the nurse is able to find out the patient's health belief model. The concept of the health belief model was originally formulated by Rosenstock (1966) to explain preventative health behaviours. This model was later adapted by Becker (1974) to explain compliance behaviour of patients on therapeutic regimens. The adapted model, summarised by Ozuna (1981: p. 2), assumes that a person is not likely to take a health action unless:

1. He believes himself susceptible to the disease in question.
2. He believes that the disease would have serious effects on his life should he contract it.
3. He is aware of certain actions that can be taken and believes that these actions reduce his likelihood of contracting the disease or reduce the severity of it.
4. He believes that the threat to him of taking the action is not as great as the threat of the disease itself.

This is the sort of in-depth information about a client which the nurse is able to acquire through the self-administration programme as a result of asking questions about drugs and illness. If the client has misconceptions about susceptibility to illness then these can be rectified by education, as can the other tenets of the health belief model. It is through giving this information that you are giving the control back to the client, because if clients have *all* (not selective) information about their drugs and their illness, they are then in a position to make informed decisions about their drugs and health. Without all the information about their drugs and illness it is not possible for clients to make informed choices. In fact it is not possible for them to make any choices whatsoever because they don't know what the options are.

The issue of control is an extremely important one. Let's take it one step further and consider what may be the end result of a patient who expects the nurse to take control over the drugs. We have all had patients say, 'You do it dear, I'm in your hands', or patients who expect the nurse to make decisions for them, 'You decide, you know what's best for me'. I think that such clients may also find it difficult to accept responsibility for their smoking habits, or how much alcohol they drink, or what they eat.

As health care professionals it is our responsibility to return the control of the patient's health back to where it belongs, the patient. We can do this by establishing a relationship with patients, by correcting any misconceptions they may have through giving education, and by encouraging and motivating them to take responsibility for making informed choices about their health. Patients may be in hospital for a very short period of their lives only, but this provides an ideal opportunity for the nurse to act as a catalyst for motivating the acceptance of personal responsibility. Such motivation is possible through the use of a self-administration programme.

## Compliance

All programmes of self-administration have been found to improve compliance with drug regimens. The reasons why self-administration improves compliance are many and complex and will be discussed fully in Chapter 6.

One simple reason to explain why compliance is improved through a self-administration programme is that the clients are educated about their drugs. What incentive do people have to take a drug if they have no understanding of the purpose of the medication, particularly if this situation is compounded by the development of a side-effect about which they have not been warned? While carrying out my own research, I was astonished by the number of patients who did not know either the name or the purpose of their drugs. An example of this poor knowledge was one patient who had been prescribed digoxin and, thinking that the purpose of this drug was to control his pain, was using it as an analgesic!

### WHAT DO PATIENTS THINK ABOUT SELF-ADMINISTRATION?

It must be obvious that all the contributors to this book are very enthusiastic about the self-administration programme. But what about the consumer? Do patients like the scheme and is there any evidence that they have actually benefited? In order to give you the patients' perspective, I have pulled out some descriptive comments from nurses who have set up self-administration programmes in a variety of different settings. I have also used some comments made by patients taken from my own research.

### What other researchers say

In their study, MacGuire and colleagues (1987) interviewed 14 patients who had self-medicated. All the patients felt that they had benefited from being a part of the self-administration programme.

Kallas (1984) noted that, in the self-administration programme she had instigated, patients commented that the programme helped them to feel independent and self-reliant and that they had benefited from the education programme and written information.

Youngren (1981) found patients in her self-medication and teaching programme to show increased pride and self-confidence as well as demonstrating good knowledge of their drug regimens.

Thompson and Ellenberg (1987) assessed the benefits of a self-administration programme which they had implemented, by using a telephone follow up. The following findings emerged:

> The patients and their families all felt that they gained a better understanding of the medications the patients were using than they ever had before. They felt furthermore, that they had a better understanding of how and when the patients were to take the medications. The vast majority of patients and families (about 90% by phone survey) felt that having a written record on discharge that included the medications and how they were supposed to be taken was extremely useful. (p. 317)

It is apparent from these comments that all the researchers felt self-medication to be beneficial to their patients.


**What the patients say**

The comments given below, which were made by patients, are taken from my own research (Bird, 1989). To set the scene I will explain how this research was carried out. All patients admitted to one ward were assessed for suitability to self-administer their drugs (using the form described in Chapter 3). If assessed to be suitable they were then randomised (by tossing a coin) into either the trial group who self-administered their drugs or the control group who had their drugs administered by nursing staff. All patients were followed up at home, by nurses using interview schedules prepared by me, within a month of being discharged from hospital. All interviews were tape recorded to enable me to check the validity of the interview and the accuracy of the interviewer.

The following comments are a selection of those made by the trial group in response to the question, 'How useful have you found the drug reminder card?'

One patient replied, 'I used to take pot luck before and didn't know what I had taken'.

Another said, 'It's a magic card isn't it? It tells you all the side-effects'.

One patient commented, 'The answer to the problem of not enough information is to give everybody a yellow card. This is the best way of giving facts using simple language, not words like "contra-indicated" or "renal impairment" which nobody can understand'.

When the trial group were asked how happy they were with the information given about their drugs one said, 'I think I got adequate information on the yellow card'.

Another said, 'On this admission I found the nurses were far more willing to talk and far more willing to explain than I've ever experienced on my previous admissions, and at the clinic I have been given no information whatsoever'.

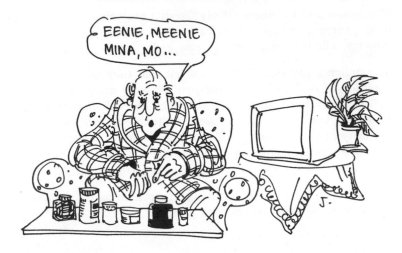

Another commented, 'Self-medication is good, you've got to carry on when you get home so you may as well start in hospital'.

Another replied, 'It's the best I've ever had'.

I think that these comments suggest that the patients benefited from the self-administration programme. Also, if you believe that the amount of information a patient receives is synonymous with patient satisfaction (Ley, 1988), then these patients must have been happy with the care they received. Keeping the customer satisfied in today's 'White Paper world', when hospitals are competing for business in the market place, is more important than ever before. If patient satisfaction is increased by self-administration of drugs in hospital, this must be an important benefit.

### THE POTENTIAL DISADVANTAGES

This would be a very biased chapter if I only discussed the benefits of a self-administration scheme so, to give you a more balanced view, the potential risks as listed in our original protocol, are outlined briefly in Table 5.1.

As you can see the list of benefits described in this chapter far outnumber the potential disadvantages. I would agree that some of the possible disadvantages (such as overdosage) have the potential to be very dangerous. However, I must also point out that during the five years that we have been operating the programme, we have experienced very few problems. We have not had anybody take an intentional overdose. Nor have we had any problems of theft – be they intentional, or unintentional with confused 'Flossie' stealing and consuming drugs unaware of the consequences.

We have certainly cared for clients who experienced difficulties with their drug regimens. I look upon this as being one of the major benefits of the programme because if you can detect problems in hospital, it is more likely that these can be rectified before the person is discharged.

**Table 5.1**  Potential risks in a self-medication programme

| Potential risk | Effect of risk |
|---|---|
| Overdose – either intentional or accidental | It must be better for this to happen in hospital where immediate action can be taken. It is impossible to predict if somebody is going to take an intentional overdose, just be thankful that the 'cry for help' has come while the person is in hospital |
| Underdosage/forgetting to take the tablet | This is definitely an advantage if you can detect this problem in hospital because it is then possible to take appropriate action, e.g. give patients more education, or devise ways to help the patient remember each dose – such as tear-off calendars |
| Theft of drugs from a patient who is self-medicating | |
| Confused patients taking drugs from self-medicating patients | |
| Non-compliance | |

Before making any change in your practice it is essential that, as a professional person, you weigh up the pros and cons and thus make an informed choice. We stress the importance of this for our patients but it is equally important for nurses. In this case getting the whole picture can be achieved through reviewing the available literature, seeking advice from experts and applying a large helping of common sense! Personally, I feel that it would be difficult for any professional reading this book to ignore the potential benefits of self-administration and, as a consequence, not to consider changing his or her practice.

# 6

# Why does self-administration improve compliance?

Whether or not patients comply with their drug regimens is a subject which concerns most health care workers. Because compliance is such an important area I felt that the topic warranted a review of the literature to establish the factors which influence adherence to treatment regimens.

I have already mentioned that self-administration programmes have been found to improve levels of compliance with drug regimens. In this chapter I will explore the reasons why this might be the case. This will be achieved firstly, through reviewing the literature and highlighting the factors which are known to improve compliance (correlates) and secondly, by noting which of the correlates are present in the self-administration scheme discussed in this book.

Before starting, I must say a few words about the actual term 'compliance' which has been criticised by many authors who have complained that it smacks of sin and discipline and implies an unequal relationship between doctors and other health care professionals and patients. I agree with this view and dislike the term myself, but for present purposes, the problems encountered in response to the term will not be discussed any further. As it is still the term most widely used, it will be employed in this book.

### Definitions

Before the factors influencing compliance can be investigated, it is important to understand what is meant by the term in relation to drug administration.

There are a number of definitions offered to explain the meaning of the term. Gill and colleagues (1981: p. 1) state: 'Compliance describes the closeness with which the patient follows his doctors or nurses instructions'. I particularly like this one because it mentions nurses. Most definitions of compliance only talk about following doctors' orders. Sackett and

Haynes (1976: p. 1) define compliance as, 'the extent to which the patient's behaviour (in terms of taking medications, following diets or executing life-style changes) coincides with the clinical prescription'.

Ley (1988: p. 54) offers a definition of non-compliance rather than compliance, and this definition is specific to medications:

> Non-compliance has been described as exhibiting one or more of the following behaviours:
> (a) not taking enough medicine;
> (b) taking too much medicine;
> (c) not observing the correct interval between doses;
> (d) not observing the correct duration of treatment;
> (e) taking additional non-prescribed medications.

Ley's description of non-compliance provides the most relevant definition for this book. This is in the main due to the fact that it is concerned solely with drug taking whereas the other definitions offered are more general, relating to compliance with all aspects of therapeutic regimes, for example diet.

It is apparent from the literature that non-compliance with therapy has been a major problem for many years and although the subject has been, and continues to be, extensively researched, no definitive answer to the problem has yet been discovered.

Koltun and Stone (1986) note that the first research concerning non-compliance appeared in 1943. From this one article in 1943, there has been a steady rise in the number of publications produced and by 1982, over 160 articles were published. These authors also comment that the fact a publication has been now produced solely for articles about compliance (*The Journal of Compliance in Health Care*) reflects the large volume of research into this subject. Several researchers describe how interest in the subject of non-compliance goes back much further than 1943 and quote from the Hippocratic writings, 'Keep watch also on the faults of patients, which makes them lie about the taking of things prescribed'. (McKercher and Rucker, 1977; Koltun and Stone, 1986; Ley, 1988).

### THE MAGNITUDE OF THE PROBLEM

When I first began looking at the statistics relating to non-compliance I was stunned at the size of the problem. Previously, I had not realised that half of the patients I was witnessing leaving hospital would not take their medication or not take it as prescribed. This did not make me feel very good about my nursing practice because obviously drug therapy is a crucial component of nursing in a medical ward, and all my nursing interventions seemed a bit pointless if patients were going to discontinue their treatment as soon as they left hospital. So how big a problem is non-compliance?

Evans and Spelman (1983), in their review of the studies which have been carried out in the field of non-compliance, estimated that almost one-half of patients do not take the drug or do not take it as prescribed, and most will stop treatment as soon as they are feeling better. Parkin and colleagues (1976) studied 130 patients, mostly acute medical cases, who were discharged from hospital. They found that 66 deviated from the drug regime prescribed on discharge.

Wandless and colleagues (1979) surveyed 81 patients aged 65 and over in their own homes. Using interviews and tablet counts they found that a deviation of more than 10% from absolute adherence to the prescription was made in 53% of all tablet counts. Feinberg (1988) reviewed the literature relating to compliance levels for patients with rheumatoid arthritis. Fifteen studies from the period 1960–1986 were reviewed. The overall compliance rates ranged from 30–78%, non-compliance rates therefore range from 22–70%.

Rashid (1982), in his study of 162 patients prescribed medication by their GPs, found that 20% failed to even cash their prescription. This he termed 'primary non-compliance'.

From the literature it would appear that non-compliance with drug regimes is a significant problem. The percentage of patients who do not comply ranges from 19–74% depending on the type of drug used. The overall average rate of non-compliance for most types of medication is 50%. Assessing the size of the problem is in itself irrelevant without measuring the cost of non-compliance to both the patient and the community.

**The cost of non-compliance**

Because non-compliance is a sizeable problem, it is logical to assume that it must also be costly in terms of human suffering and financial expenditure. Researchers have tended to concern themselves with different aspects of the 'cost'. For example, the cost which has concerned Haynes and his colleagues (1987) is the failed potential of modern medicine. They state (p. 156):

> If true tragedy lies in the failure to achieve that which can be achieved, then non-compliance is a tragic flaw in our efforts to reap the benefits of treatment that work when they are taken.

This sounds more like a piece from Shakespeare than the writings of twentieth century authors, however their point is clear and I do agree with the content even if it is somewhat dramatic.

Falvo and colleagues (1980) also note that treatment failure is a likely consequence of patients not adhering to their drug regimes. They go on to suggest that this may involve the patient in further unnecessary diagnostic procedures and treatment.

Some authors have assessed the cost of non-compliance in financial terms as well as in terms of treatment failure. For example Gill and colleagues (1981) note that non-compliance is a significant drain to the community on both health and financial grounds and patients who are not taking their drugs are more likely to be readmitted to hospital, or will at the very least need to visit their GP.

Ley (1988) reviewed the work of some American researchers who estimated the cost of non-compliance in dollars. The United States Department of Health and Human Services estimated that there would be some 75 million prescriptions per year for drugs in which non-compliance could cause problems. The rate of non-compliance was assumed to be 40% and therefore it was possible to estimate the cost. The cost of each outcome was, in 1979, estimated as follows: extra prescription – $7, visit to doctor – $15, day in hospital – $250, workday lost – $45. The results are summarised in Table 6.1. These findings suggest that non-compliance is extremely expensive. As well as these financial costs non-compliance is also expensive in terms of the human costs of suffering and inconvenience caused to patients and their families.

**Table 6.1**   Estimated costs of non-compliance with regimens for ten common drug classes

| Source of cost | Estimated occurrence (%) | Estimated cost (1979) (millions of US dollars) |
|---|---|---|
| Unnecessary prescription refill | 10.0–20.0 | 21.0–42.0 |
| One additional physician visit | 5.0–10.0 | 22.5–45.0 |
| One additional workday lost | 5.0–10.0 | 67.5–135.0 |
| Two additional workdays lost | 5.0–10.0 | 135.0–270.0 |
| Hospitalisation: | | |
| One day | 0.25–0.5 | 18.75–37.5 |
| Two days | 0.50–1.0 | 75.0–150.0 |
| Three days | 0.25–0.5 | 56.25–112.5 |
| Total | | 396.0–792.0 |

**A REVIEW OF THE FACTORS WHICH MAY INFLUENCE COMPLIANCE**

Bearing in mind the enormous cost of non-compliance, it is appropriate to ask, 'Why don't patients comply with therapeutic regimes?'

Why would someone who has gone to the trouble and expense of seeking out a physician, of undertaking arduous or uncomfortable tests and other diagnostic procedures, and of purchasing drugs and devices on the advice of the physician, then fail to follow the recommendations?

(Stone, 1979: p. 22)

In this section, some of the reasons offered by researchers, to explain why patients do not comply with treatment, will be reviewed. The many studies which have looked at the factors contributing to non-compliance do not agree which ones are predictive of non-compliance.

> The factors concerned in failure to comply with therapeutic regimens are complex. Rarely does a patient default for one single reason but rather because of a multiplicity of reasons that interact to produce a state of affairs in which compliance is difficult. The approach must be based above all on an awareness of the diverse nature of the problem and must seek primarily to prevent it. (O'Hanrahan and O'Malley, 1981)

This statement is borne out by the findings of Haynes and colleagues (1979). They reviewed the interventions which, it has been suggested, enhance compliance – and found that a single intervention of any sort was insufficient to improve long term compliance.

The fact that failure to comply is usually due to a number of reasons is relevant to health care professionals. This is because part of our role is to try and make compliance the easy option and, to achieve this, we need to be aware of the variety of interventions which may have to be incorporated into the patient's care. Harper (1984) in her study of self-care medication behaviours in the elderly is more specific and lists four factors found to relate to non-compliance:

- Inadequate knowledge about medication and its administration.
- Inconsistent self-care behaviours related to medication administration.
- Limited time and involvement spent in the provider-patient interaction promoting individual responsibility for self-care.
- Lack of education programmes tailored to the learning needs of the elderly.

### The effects of drug education

Educating patients about their drugs and checking that the information has been understood is mentioned by several researchers to be one method of improving compliance (Harper, 1984). Macdonald and colleagues (1977) studied the effects of drug education (described as counselling by the researchers) on medication errors in 165 elderly patients who had been discharged from hospital. They found a considerable increase in patients taking their tablets correctly in the counselled group. The research of Kellaway and McCrae (1979) also demonstrated that patient counselling can improve levels of compliance with drug treatment.

In the majority of British studies which have investigated the effects of drug education on compliance, the pharmacist and/or the doctor have been the providers of this education. However, it would appear to make no difference which health professional counsels patients about their drugs. Edwards and Pathy (1984) evaluated the effects of counselling about medication by different professional groups, doctors, nurses or pharmacists. It was found that formal counselling resulted in an appreciable improvement in compliance regardless of profession. Personally, I feel that a team approach is the best way to ensure that patients receive adequate information about their drugs, and doctors, nurses, and pharmacists should all participate in providing and reinforcing this essential information.

O'Hanrahan and O'Malley (1981) also mention that explaining the purpose of the treatment to the patient is a strategy to improve compliance. These authors also note that forewarning the client about possible side-effects can improve compliance. The question of whether or not to tell patients about the potential side-effects of their treatment is a controversial one and the medical profession frequently appears to disagree over this issue. Meichenbaum and Turk (1987) quote a survey of physicians carried out by Ascione and Raven (1975) which revealed that 75% of physicians did not wish patients to be told about the potential side-effects of prescribed medication.

The general feeling appears to be that patients will automatically develop symptoms if they know what the side-effects are, and having developed them are more likely to stop treatment. There is, however, no evidence to support this 'general feeling' held by some medical staff. In actual fact the research suggests the opposite; patients are more likely to stop taking their drugs if they are not told about possible side-effects. For example:

> It is mainly unexpected and alarming side effects of treatment that patients offer as reason for stopping treatment. Most side effects can be anticipated and forewarning patients of their potential occurrence has not been demonstrated to affect either their incidence or patients' nonadherence. (Blackwell, 1973: p. 148)

Ridout and colleagues (1986) assessed how many patients were aware of the possible unwanted effects associated with their drugs. (This was part of a study to investigate the need for drug information leaflets.) These researchers found that of the 154 people questioned, 112 (72%) knew of no side-effects which could result from their medicine.

## Complexity of drug regimens

Many researchers have examined the effect of the number of different drugs prescribed and the number of doses upon compliance. For example Ozuna (1981) notes that:

> Patients on complex regimens are less likely to comply than those on simple ones. Persons taking more pills more frequently tend not to comply as well as those taking a single daily dose of medication. (p. 1)

Hulka and colleagues (1975) found that errors increased with the number of medicines taken. The work of Parkin and colleagues (1976) agrees with the findings of Hulka *et al.* and these researchers also found that patients did worse if they needed more doses each day. Stone (1979) was more specific and reported that the error or rate of non-adherence was 15% when patients were asked to take one drug. This increases to 25% on two or three medications, and to 35% if more than five drugs are prescribed.

### The doctor/patient relationship

The quality of this relationship as a method of improving compliance has been considered by many researchers. In Britain it appears to have been general practitioners who have been most interested in exploring this relationship. An example of research carried out by GPs in this area is the work of Ettlinger and Freeman (1981) who hypothesised that close identification with a doctor leads to improved drug compliance. They tested this hypothesis through studying 119 patients in the community. Their findings demonstrated that compliance with the prescription was strongly associated with whether the patient thought that he knew the prescribing doctor well. Two other GPs, Graham and Suppree (1979), also suggest that the good doctor/patient relationship found in general practice may contribute to improved levels of compliance. These authors cite the work of Cherney and colleagues (1967) who found that penicillin prescribed to children was taken more accurately if they and their parents were seen by their usual practitioner rather than a partner.

If we accept that the relationship between the patient and the doctor or other health practitioner may improve compliance, then it is important to isolate the characteristics of this relationship which apparently contribute to improved compliance. O'Hanrahan and O'Malley (1981) note that the most important features of the doctor/patient relationship which influence compliance are: 'the extent to which patient's expectations are met; his level of satisfaction with the visit; and the level of communication between the two' (p. 299).

Some of these findings are confirmed by Ley (1988) who notes that although several researchers have investigated the relationship between therapist and patient in connection with compliance, too few studies have been carried out for any generalisation to be made. However, he does state that there are three characteristics of the patient/therapist interaction which have been shown to be associated with compliance. These are (Ley, 1988: p. 68):

- Patients' satisfaction.
- Patients' expectations being met.
- Level of supervision by the therapist.

Falvo and colleagues (1980) investigated the relationship of doctor behaviour to patient compliance. Their findings suggested that the patient's perception of the doctor's behaviour was important. If the patient perceived that the doctor was giving adequate information about treatment, and was considering the patient's concerns when prescribing this treatment, he or she would be more likely to comply.

The therapist/patient relationship appears to be crucial to compliance. Although researchers cannot agree on the exact characteristics of the relationship which affect compliance, they do agree that it has a part to play.

### Customised care and encouraging patient participation

Several researchers have noted the importance of customising care for each client as a method of improving compliance. Tailoring the care for each individual is likely to improve patient satisfaction, and thus compliance, because the health care professional is spending quality time with the person, giving the person information which is relevant to his or her previous knowledge base, and the stage of the illness.

Following on from customising care, some authors recommend contingency contracting as a way of both encouraging patient participation and improving compliance. Kosnar (1987) defines contingency contracting as a mutual and negotiable working agreement between the nurse and the client. She notes that contracting for care improves the patients' level of satisfaction by allowing them actively to participate in the restoring of their health. Zangari and Duffy (1980) mention that as well as improving patient satisfaction, contracting also increases nurse satisfaction through helping to prevent clients from taking on the 'sick role', avoiding undue dependence and helping them to retain control.

### Physical difficulties

Several researchers have noted that physical difficulties commonly cause problems with drug taking, Todd (1981); Gibb (1985); Punton (1985); and Hall (1981). I am sure that all health care professionals have cared for patients who are unable to open child resistant bottles. As it is routine to supply drugs with these types of closure, it is not surprising that a significant number of patients will be unable to open them and thus be unable to comply.

### Age

Physical difficulties are more likely to be a problem for the elderly. However, there appears to be an assumption made by many health care workers that there is a correlation between age itself and non-compliance. The majority of the researchers who have studied compliance with drug regimens have therefore concentrated on those in the over 65 age group. There is very little evidence, however, to support the assumption that the elderly are less likely to comply than younger patients.

Ley (1988) notes that elderly people might be less compliant as a result of poor eyesight and hearing, poor memory, and the fact that they are more likely to be living alone. Following this comment, Ley reviews ten studies which assessed levels of compliance with drug regimes in patients over 60. The findings of these studies demonstrated that compliance rates in the elderly range widely as they do in other age groups. The mean compliance was 51% which compares favourably with estimates of overall compliance in other age groups.

> Thus non-compliance is a problem in the treatment of the elderly as well as in the treatment of younger groups, but it does not seem to be a significantly greater problem.                     (Ley, 1988: p. 65)

O'Hanrahan and O'Malley (1981) agree with Ley's conclusions and mention that elderly individuals who are confused may need supervision but otherwise elderly patients are no less likely to be non-compliant than younger ones.

Sackett and Haynes (1976) carried out what is probably the most extensive review of studies relating to compliance. They reviewed 37 studies concerned with compliance and the elderly. Only seven of these found that compliance was greater among the young; 30 found that there was no relationship between age and compliance. Wandless and colleagues (1979) found no significant relationship between age and compliance in their study of 81 patients aged 65 and over.

The elderly have received a great deal of sustained attention over the years from researchers in the field of compliance. It would appear however, from the literature, that although they are more prone to the physical disabilities which could lead to practical problems with drug taking, the elderly are no less likely to comply than their younger counterparts.


## The health belief model

A number of researchers have found that the patient's own health belief model is a significant predictor of whether or not he or she is likely to comply. Cameron and Gregor (1987) note:

> That a patient's perspective will determine his decision to comply is substantiated in the health belief model, one of the most frequently researched explanations of compliance. (p. 673)

Meichenbaum and Turk (1987) state:

> Patients hold many beliefs about their health and about the potential efficacy of any proposed treatment action. Sometimes the patients beliefs are based on misconceptions, faulty information, negative distortions and cultural myths. In addition, patient feelings of fear, guilt, fatalism, shame, and "paralyses of will" can also contribute to treatment non-adherence. (p. 46)

Ozuna (1981) also suggests that the health belief model could offer useful guidelines for developing health education programmes for patients prescribed long-term drug therapy. Ozuna gives the example of a person who has suffered one or maybe two epileptic fits and says that if he does not believe that he is susceptible to further seizures, then he is unlikely to take medication to prevent recurring fits.

Ley (1988) notes that the variables of the health belief model, namely the patient's perceived vulnerability, seriousness of illness and efficacy of treatment, appear to be important determinants of compliance.

### HOW MAY LEVELS OF COMPLIANCE BE IMPROVED?

We are now getting to the crux of the matter, what can we actually do in order to improve our patients' levels of compliance with their drug regimens? Don't get too excited here because although many investigators have studied factors that contribute to compliance, few have been able to agree which ones are predictive of non-compliance. Consequently the suggestions for improving compliance tend to be based on the authors' own research findings rather than from a review of all available research. So for the purpose of this book I have reviewed a great deal of the literature and have produced the following list which consists of the factors which are most commonly noted by other researchers.

### Recommendations

Newcomer and Anderson (1974) recommended that a combined drug self-administration system and teaching programme should be introduced for hospital patients. The idea behind this scheme was to encourage patients to become involved in their own treatment regimen prior to discharge. Clark-Mahoney (1984) also found that a programme of self-medication and teaching for hospital patients improved compliance.

Several researchers (e.g. Kellaway and McCrae, 1979, and Macdonald et al., 1977) noted that educating patients about their medications is a method of improving compliance. Hermann and colleagues (1978) recommend that verbal counselling should be supplemented with written information. The American Society of Hospital Pharmacists (1976) stated that the information given to patients should include the following:

- Name of drug.
- Intended use and expected action.
- Rate, dosage, form, administration schedule.
- Specific direction for preparation.
- Specific direction for administration.
- Precautions to be observed during use.
- Common side-effects.

- Proper storage conditions.
- Potential interactions.
- Prescription refill information.
- Action to take if dose missed.
- Any other specific information required particular to the patient.

O'Hanrahan and O'Malley (1981) suggest the following as a strategy to improve compliance. The regimen should be kept as simple as possible, avoiding excessive numbers of doses or preparations. The doctor must ensure that the patient understands the details of the regimen, the need for treatment and the importance of any likely side-effects.

Haynes and colleagues (1987) are among the few authors who have carried out an extensive review of the literature pertaining to interventions to improve compliance. Haynes suggests that the following list of actions may improve compliance with medication:

- Keep the prescription as simple as possible.
- Give clear, preferably written instructions on the treatment regimen.
- Give reminders in the form of prescribing medication to fit in with the patient's daily schedule.
- Give rewards such as recognising the patient's efforts to comply.
- Involve the patient's spouse or other partner.

Wade and Bowling (1986) also based their recommendations on the findings from other researchers in the field of compliance. These authors advise that the following (very comprehensive) list of recommendations should be incorporated into drug regimes to improve compliance (see Wade and Bowling, 1986: p. 50).

1. Keep the number of drugs and administration times to an essential minimum.
2. Aim for the most pleasant form of presentation possible and keep to the same form of presentation throughout treatment.
3. Work out drug regimens to fit in with the individual's daily routine and supportive help as available.
4. Explain the purpose of the medication. Explain any possible side-effects and action to take.
5. Explain dosage instructions.
6. Use a suitable container, checking that the patient can handle it. Use large bottles so that labelling can be adequate.
7. Label clearly in large letters, preferably type. Include labels on the reverse side of the container to contain additional instructions.
8. Supply instruction sheet explaining drug regimen.
9. Ensure that the patient knows what to do about further supplies of medications.
10. Ensure that the patient knows who to contact in case of any queries or difficulties.

11. Review prescriptions and progress regularly in longer-term care situations.
12. Explain to the patient the importance of disposing of all unused drugs.
13. Ensure that the patient can repeat essentials of instructions in his/her own words.
14. Ensure that all those concerned with the patient's care are aware of what each other is doing and what instructions have been issued.

**Summary**

A review of the books and articles relating to compliance reveals that non-compliance is expensive in both financial terms and in terms of human suffering. The subject of compliance has been extensively researched and a number of factors which may influence it have been isolated. Although not all researchers are able to agree on which of these may be predictive of non-compliance, certain common factors do emerge, which, when grouped together form the basis of recommendations to help improve levels of compliance. These recommendations include:

- Giving patients adequate information both about their illness and about the rationale behind treatment.
- Giving patients an explanation of the purpose of their medications and details of the regime including possible side-effects.
- Simplifying the prescription and fitting it in with the individual's daily routine.
- Checking understanding.
- Using a suitable container.
- The giving of rewards such as recognising the patient's efforts to comply.
- Involving the patient's spouse or other partner.

An average of 50% of patients do not take their drugs as prescribed and, despite extensive research over the past 40 years, these levels of non-compliance have not improved. One of the reasons suggested to explain this continuing high level of non-compliance is that health care professionals remain unaware of the basic compliance management principles.

As we have now looked at some of the factors which influence compliance, let's now discuss why self-administration of drugs is likely to improve compliance.

### WHICH CORRELATES OF COMPLIANCE CAN BE FOUND IN A PROGRAMME OF SELF-ADMINISTRATION?

In the previous section of this chapter, the factors which are known to contribute to improved levels of compliance have been outlined. It may now be of value to determine which of these factors are present in self-administration programmes. In order to do this, the factors which have been found to improve patient compliance will be used as headings. Beneath each heading it should be possible, through reviewing the literature pertaining to self-medication, to determine which factors known to improve compliance are present in both our own and other authors' programmes of self-administration.

### Giving adequate information

Giving patients information has been found by several researchers to be a method of improving compliance (George, 1987; Association of the British Pharmaceutical Industry, 1987b). This information should include the name and purpose of the drug, administration details and possible side-effects. The verbal information should be supplemented with written information.

All the systems of self-medication described in the literature included an education programme. For example Youngren (1981), describing the system of self-medication in her unit for patients with chronic lung disease, states:

> After describing each prescribed drug, its expected action, and side-effects, the nurse gave the patient a medication handout summarising this information, the drug's appearance, purpose, dosage and schedule, and what to do if side effects occur. (p. 22)

In our own programme of self-administration we give each patient verbal information which is backed up with written information in the form of the drug reminder card. The information is tailored to suit each patient and care is taken to ensure that the information is given using language the patient can understand, and delivered at an appropriate stage of the patient's illness.

### Simplifying the prescription

Many researchers in the field of compliance suggest that simplifying drug regimes may lead to improved patient adherence (Haynes *et al.*, 1987; Hulka *et al.*, 1975; Ozuna, 1981; Parkin *et al.*, 1976; Stone, 1979).

It has been noted that a programme of self-administration may encourage the medical staff to rationalise and simplify the drug regimen. For example Hursey (1985) implemented a programme of self-medication in an elderly care unit. She noted that simplification of each patient's medication regime was an important part of the programme.

In my own area it has certainly become part of the normal routine, within the self-administration scheme, to simplify the drug regimen. This is carried out by the whole multidisciplinary team working together in order to help make it easier for patients to take their drugs.

**Practical considerations**

Several researchers have noted that many patients had difficulty opening drug containers and reading labels, and that this means reduced compliance (Hall, 1981; Kendrick and Bayne, 1982; Potter, 1981). Other authors suggested that fitting the drug regimen into the patient's daily routine increased the chance of compliance (Wade and Bowling, 1986).

Most authors of self-medication articles mentioned that, because patients were responsible for taking their own drugs in hospital, any problems they might experience with using conventional containers would be observed and appropriate action taken. For example, Thompson and Ellenberg (1987) found that the physical difficulties experienced by patients due to the design of the containers, proved to be a challenging and rewarding part of the self-medication programme. In this programme each patient was assessed, and adaptive equipment which best fitted the individual's needs was devised.

Kallas (1984) reported that self-medication enabled nurses to recognise patients who were unable to use conventional containers. Hatch and Tapley (1982) found it was necessary to include the following measures to ensure that patients were able to take their drugs: large labels on drug containers, colour coding or even Braille labels if the patient was blind.

Our self-administration programme involves assessing patients for practical problems (such as opening bottles or reading labels). If a particular client does have a problem, then appropriate measures can be used (such as putting larger print on labels or using bottles with non-childproof closures).

Self-administration may be a useful method of helping patients to become accustomed to fitting their drug taking into their daily routine. For example, MacGuire and colleagues (1987) found that using mealtimes on the drug labels could help patients to take their drugs correctly. Kallas (1984) reported that several patients who had self-medicated commented that the programme helped them to establish a medication schedule they could readily continue at home.

We encourage patients to try and establish a routine whilst in hospital, and nurses always question the patient to find out when they would normally take medication at home before completing their drug reminder card.

**Patient participation/retaining control**

Allowing patients to participate in their care and retain control of their health is likely to contribute to increased levels of patient satisfaction and understanding. This, in turn, is likely to improve compliance (Zangari and Duffy, 1980; Cameron and Gregor, 1987; Kosnar, 1987).

A programme of self-medication automatically ensures patient participation because it requires patients to be responsible for and administer their own medications. Several authors have noted the importance of this feature. For example, Scriven (1987) found that self-medication encouraged patients to feel they had control over what happened to them in hospital. Punton (1985) noted that patients who had self-medicated were able to maintain a sense of responsibility for themselves. Thompson and Ellenberg (1987) mentioned that a system in which patients can manage their medications gives them direct involvement in their own care. Youngren (1981) reported that patients involved in a self-medication treatment programme showed increased pride and self-confidence. Hatch and Tapley (1982) noted that a system of self-medication gave patients greater independence.

### Involving the patient's spouse or significant others

Including the patient's relatives in the drug education programme has been noted by Haynes *et al.* (1987) to be a method of improving compliance. Relatives are often involved in the care when patients are self-medicating. For example, Gibb (1985) included any relatives who had regular contact with the patient in the self-medication programme she instigated. Youngren (1981) found that the patient's family could be useful in reinforcing the information given by the nurse.

Relatives are automatically included in our programme if both the patient and their family desire this. It is quite normal for patients themselves to include their relatives by showing them their drug reminder cards and the other documentation from the programme. Frequently the whole family then discusses the patient's drugs and we hear comments such as 'I never knew what that was for' and 'It does make it clear doesn't it, Bert?'. If the client normally has the medication administered by a relative or friend at home and is happy for this to continue, then we will, as a matter of routine, give the relevant education to this person.

### Customising care

Customising the programme of education for the individual patient, including pacing the amount of information given, is a method of improving both compliance and satisfaction (Meichenbaum and Turk, 1987; Harper, 1984).

All the programmes of self-administration described in the literature involve individualised patient assessment and teaching. For example, Hursey (1985) notes that self-medicating patients are counselled by a pharmacist to assess their understanding of the medication and to try and predict potential problems. Baxendale and colleagues (1978) mention that when a patient is self-medicating, 'the emphasis changes from taking medicine at ward round times to following a timetable suitable for the patient . . .'. Thompson and Ellenberg (1987) gave their self-medicating patients a discharge booklet which contained a section on medication. This booklet was customised to meet the patient's needs and included information about the purpose of the drugs, administration details and potential side-effects. Bream (1985) states:

Self-medicating patients were taught about their drugs in a series of three flexible periods, enabling each programme to be patient-designed.

## IN CONCLUSION

Although somewhat sparse, the literature relating to self-medication reveals that many of the interventions found to improve patient compliance and satisfaction are an integral part of self-medication programmes. The intervention present in self-medication programmes include:

- Ensuring that patients receive both written and verbal drug information.
- Simplifying the prescription.
- Customising the programme to suit the individual's requirements and knowledge base.
- Observing for and adapting to meet the patient's practical needs.
- Encouraging patient participation.
- Including patients' relatives in the programme.

Another factor found to be a correlate of compliance is the doctor/patient relationship. There is no direct connection between this relationship and self-administration, but what is apparent is that self-administration necessitates the health care practitioner spending more time with self-medicating patients. This in itself may be a correlate of compliance.

The fact that programmes of self-administration improve compliance is indisputable. Although many of the researchers cannot definitely agree on the specific factors which improve compliance, there is sufficient evidence to demonstrate that many of the correlates of compliance are present in a self-administration scheme.

# 7

# The pharmacist's perspective on self-administration of drugs

This chapter will provide an overview of the pharmacist's involvement in all stages of the self-administration programme from planning to introduction and implementation. The main areas where pharmacist advice is essential are covered – including storage of medication and patient counselling. Within these topics there is a brief discussion of some of the methods employed to address these issues.

The self-administration process involves a number of health care professionals and it is vital that procedures and policies are produced. Those that require input from the pharmacist are discussed.

With the introduction of any new system there are often problems that may arise and self-administration is no exception. The problems that are likely to be encountered are reviewed along with a discussion of potential solutions, although it should be stressed that neither is an exhaustive list.

The chapter provides practical details and information that could be used by any health care professional involved in the design and implementation of a self-administration programme. It needs to be stressed that the methods and solutions described in this chapter work well for the self-administration programme at the John Radcliffe in Oxford. That does not necessarily mean, however, that they will translate into another setting. Rather, they should be used as a framework when local policies and procedures are designed.

## PATIENTS' KNOWLEDGE OF AND COMPLIANCE WITH THEIR MEDICATION

The Royal Pharmaceutical Society of Great Britain periodically runs a 'dump' campaign where patients are encouraged to return unused and unwanted medicines. The quantity returned is revealing about the wastage of medication, and a proportion of this wastage will be related to patients not fulfilling their prescriptions.

Compliance and non-compliance of patients with their medication are terms used when discussing the patient completing the prescription supplied

84

by the doctor. Both terms imply an all or none response, suggesting that the patient who complies fulfils 100% of the prescription while the patient who does not comply fails to take any. Realities may not be as clear cut as this, however. Many patients will fall between these two extremes, either due to genuine lapses or through deliberate decision not to take their medication. The outcome of either problem can be serious. For example, the patient who takes all his or her medicines prior to an outpatient appointment will be at risk of overdose and subsequent side-effects. Alternatively the patient who stops taking their medication can suffer just as serious consequences with a loss of therapeutic effect (Walshie and Dixon, 1986).

It is very difficult to assess the degree of patient compliance with their medication. Tablet counts have traditionally been regarded as a simple and convenient method of establishing compliance. However, there are now suspicions being raised that between 30% and 50% of patients who return the correct numbers of tablets can still be non-compliant. Tablet counts are also claimed to be unreliable and inaccurate, with their use in monitoring drug compliance in clinical trials being called into question (Pullar et al., 1989).

New ways to try and measure compliance involve the use of microprocessors located in the cap of the medicine bottle. Each time the bottle is opened a medication event is recorded and the number of openings can be related to the number of tablets that should have been taken (Cramer et al., 1989). This is not without its problems as the microprocessor cannot take into account the number of tablets actually removed at each opening. For a small number of drugs it is possible to measure their concentration in the blood of patients taking these drugs and this is known as therapeutic drug monitoring. This allows clinical decisions on whether the dose needs increasing or decreasing, if so by how much, whether the drug is still effective or whether the adverse events the patient is experiencing are related to the drug. Also, measuring the concentration of the drug will establish whether the patient has been taking the drug recently and therefore exhibiting compliance. This is still far from ideal, however, as the serum concentration will not quantify the degree of compliance.

A group of workers have developed the use of a phenobarbital tracer to assess compliance (Feely et al., 1987). They measure the level of the phenobarbital in the patient's blood and with this method they are able to get a good picture of compliance. In a comparison of the two methods only 13% of non-compliance episodes identified by the phenobarbital tracer method were identified by tablet counts (Pullar et al., 1988).

One of the ways to help alleviate the problem of patients not taking their medication is the use of compliance aids. These are directed particularly towards patients with problems in remembering instructions or directions. The compliance aids are often designed so that the patient's medication for each day and even each administration time (e.g. breakfast, dinner) can easily be obtained. They usually only hold one week's supply at a time and so supervision of their filling is required, although there is no reason why this should not be done by the patient's community pharmacist. Another problem is that the compliance aids can be difficult to manipulate and this can further limit the population they can be used in (Cowderoy and Coker, 1987). Compliance aids available include the Dosett, Medidose and Doseaid – and there will undoubtedly be others as technology improves.

There may be a number of reasons why patients do not adhere to their regimen. As the complexity of their prescribed medication regimen increases so the greater the likelihood of non-compliance. The increase in the frequency of administration above twice daily may start to lead to problems (Pullar *et al.*, 1988). The use of clear instructions along with an unambiguous label is vital to ensure that the patient understands the prescription. The patient may not be able actually to swallow the tablets or capsules, or may find the formulation unpalatable. Just as important is the ability of the patient to open the container, which must be ascertained. Someone who cannot open a medication container will not take the medication. There may also be side-effects related to some medications that will actively discourage patients from taking them regularly. An example of such is drowsiness, and patients should be warned to avoid driving with some antihistamines, and taking alcohol with metronidazole for example (Cowderoy and Coker, 1987). All these issues are important and must be addressed to establish why a patient is not complying with his or her prescribed regimen.

### Information

The provision of information is a vital part of the prescribing process to ensure that compliance with the medication regimen is adhered to. Verbal information will encourage compliance and addition of written information may provide further improvement (Colcher *et al.*, 1972; Dodds, 1986). The responsibility for provision of information is often shared between the pharamacist, doctor and nurse with a different emphasis from each of the professionals involved. The doctor is more likely to inform about side-effects and duration of therapy, while the pharmacist may concentrate on the best way to take medication, how frequently and how much each time (McMahon *et al.*, 1987). There are problems in that patients are seen by the doctor, and are told something about their prescriptions which are then presented to the pharmacist. The quandary for the pharmacist is to know exactly what the doctor has told each patient, particularly if the patient has already forgotten what the doctor said. The continuity and concordance of the information is essential to avoid confusing patients and to ensure that the information given by the doctor is reinforced rather than contradicted (Drugs and Therapeutic Bulletin, 1981).

Ways to overcome this have included the provision of written information with the medication. This could be a locally designed leaflet for use with specific drugs (Dodds, 1986; George *et al.*, 1983). The importance of a well designed information leaflet cannot be stressed enough to ensure that complete understanding by the patient is obtained whilst avoiding confusion. The information provided must be concise, brief and comprehensible. It should never be seen as replacing the vital role all health care professionals have in their verbal communication with the patient (George, 1987).

There is concern that increasing patients' awareness about side-effects of their medication will increase their reporting of these. So far, however, increased awareness does not appear to have led to a rise in reporting of side-effects (BMJ, 1980). Inclusion of patient information leaflets led to an improvement in the patients' satisfaction with their treatment.

Information on certain medication such as steroids or anticoagulants has been available for some time but has often been given in the form of warning cards (Sloan, 1984).

The desire to improve patients' knowledge about their medication has led the Association of the British Pharmaceutical Industry to recommend that information leaflets be included in all medications supplied by the industry (*Lancet*, 1987a). There are still worries about the type of information that will appear on these leaflets (*Lancet*, 1987b) and, already, there are reports of confusion among patients caused by the information leaflet present with the medication (Lowen and Tejani, 1991). However the general view is that there is a definite need for patient information leaflets in one form or another (Higson, 1991). Certain simple information is provided by some disease trusts – for example the British Heart Foundation produces excellent leaflets on angina, heart attacks and other cardiac problems.

It appears that, despite all the developments within health care, we still have a long way to go to improve patients' understanding of their medication. Schemes which lead to improving this must be beneficial to the patient and an already overburdened health service. Self-administration programmes bring the elements of verbal and written information to the patient counselling interview. This must improve the likelihood that patients will retain the vital information that is imparted to them in such a setting. Ultimately, this will lead to a greater understanding on the patients' part which should lead to improved patient compliance.

## PROBLEMS TO BE ADDRESSED IN SELF-ADMINISTRATION

When introducing a self-administration programme before procedures are finalised there are a number of problems that need to be addressed before general acceptance is obtained. Some of the problems encountered within the pharmacy department are described and some possible solutions are also discussed. If certain problems cannot be overcome, redesign or alteration of the programme may be necessary.

## Storage of medication

This is the biggest headache for the chief pharmacist in the hospital when the idea of a self-medication scheme is introduced. This person in liaison with the senior nurse in charge of the ward is responsible for the safe storage of medication while the patient is in hospital. Therefore it may be stipulated that the medication is stored in a locked receptacle – for example, locks could be fitted to the patient's locker. Alternatively, a specially designed trolley could be purchased or the existing trolley modified. These situations are not without their problems for the patient population as discussed later.

Where an open system is decided upon, with patients storing their own medication in their locker (out of sight), then the type of medication used in the programme may be limited. Patients on controlled drugs are likely (certainly in the initial stages of a programme) to be excluded where such a system operates.

## Controlled drugs

Self-administration programmes take careful planning prior to their introduction which will be a complex process. Inclusion of controlled drugs during the initial stages will complicate matters further. Problems such as recording the ordering and receipt of controlled drugs, their administration to patients and the recording of the quantity on the ward at any one time, must all be investigated carefully to ensure that the legal requirements for storage and handling of controlled drugs are met. There are no easy answers to this problem and any solution has to be locally agreed after careful discussion.

Controlled drugs should not be omitted from self-administration programmes, but they should only be introduced once the programme has been running for long enough to resolve any teething problems.

## Dispensing time

In most pharmacy departments the supply of drugs to the wards matches a list of drugs normally kept on the wards (so called 'ward stock drugs'). The ward stock drugs are usually in containers of 50 to 100 tablets, with no directions on, and are totally inappropriate for self-administration. When a patient is prescribed a drug that is not on the ward stock list, a bottle is dispensed from the pharmacy for that individual patient. Usually, 70–80% of the medication a patient receives is available on the ward with the remainder being dispensed individually. In the self-administration programme, 100% of a participating patient's medication will have to be dispensed from the pharmacy with the patient's name and the directions of how to take the medicine on the bottle. This could lead to a five-fold increase in the workload of the pharmacy department if self-administration was being implemented across the whole hospital. As a result, the pharmacy department may well put the brake on the progress of self-administration and may in fact refuse to sanction the programme. That is an extreme view and what is more likely is that a degree of control may be imposed on the spread of self-administration. This may include a limit on the number of patients on a ward that can be in the self-administration programme at any one time. Alternatively the limit may be imposed on the number of wards that can participate in the programme, or there may even be a combination of the two with limited numbers of patients on specified wards. This will also be influenced by the type of patient population and their drug therapy on the self-administration wards.

One alternative may be to use the patients' own medication that they bring into hospital with them. However patients' own drugs are often mixed up and removed from the original container so that the label on the bottle does not correspond with its contents. This situation is far from ideal and although extremely useful in identifying patients' medication is dangerous to make use of in a self-administration programme. In Oxford, we do make use of the drugs that patients bring in from home but only after the ward pharmacist has checked that the drugs are what the label states they are and that they are in date. If the pharmacist is satisfied then he or she will attach a sticky label which states that the medication has been checked.

Some of the workload can be reduced by dispensing more than a week's supply for patients on self-administration. This would avoid their tablets being re-dispensed when they are discharged home and speeds their discharge from the hospital as they don't have to wait for a doctor to write their prescription. This also reduces the pressure put on the pharmacy department through urgent last minute requests for take-out prescriptions.

### Staffing levels

If the workload is to be increased in the pharmacy department then pharmacy management may insist on an increase in staffing levels to accommodate this. There is no easy solution to this problem although limitation of self-administration may allow the extra work to be absorbed into the existing staffing structure. Use of a pilot study to identify the exact workload will be invaluable in this setting.

There are funds available for quality initiatives in the health service, and self-administration should be regarded as introducing further quality to patient care. Applications for funding from this source may prove fruitful and help to address the problem of staffing.

### Opposition to self-administration

Self-administration involves co-operation of a number of health care professionals and there may be a group of individuals who are against the programme. Examples might include pharmacists, as suggested above under storage of medication, time and staffing. In addition, medical staff may well not wish others to inform patients about their medication. Neither should it be forgotten that the nursing staff may not wish to take on the responsibility of a self-medication programme or may not themselves have the time for such a programme. How can these problems be overcome? Usually, if the programme is being blocked by any members of the health care team, it is due to lack of knowledge about the benefits of such a scheme. Initial involvement of all relevant members of the health care team should help to reduce opposition to change.

**Generic prescribing and the community**

When drugs are dispensed in the hospital generic substitution occurs. A drug prescribed by a trade name (e.g. Brufen) will be labelled and dispensed as the generic form (e.g. ibuprofen). The generic form may well be different in appearance to the trade name form. This is not a problem within the hospital where the tablet is attached to a medication card or the patient is shown the appearance of the tablet. However when patients are discharged and visit their own doctor who issues a new prescription then problems can arise. The pharmacist in the community must dispense the form requested by the doctor. If the trade name is used then this is what must be dispensed and if a generic is prescribed there is no guarantee that the pharmacist in the community will stock the same generic form that is used in the hospital. There is potential for confusion for patients once they have returned to the community as their tablets may change appearance completely. To reduce this, patients must have this situation explained to them so that they can question any change in appearance with the pharmacist in the community. A medication record card is very useful and patients must be encouraged to take this to their doctor and along to the pharmacy where their prescription is dispensed. This will ensure that if a tablet of different appearance is used it can be attached to the card to replace the original (see Chapter 4).

**The prescription chart**

The prescription chart currently available within the hospital may not help the self-administration programme. Often, drug administration times do not correspond with the times when patients will take their medication at home. They can be regarded as quite unsociable particularly where they are already printed on the prescription chart (e.g. 6.00 AM for the first dose in the morning). Where the times are written in after the medication is prescribed, then the times can be set to accommodate the patient's lifestyle. The design of a new prescription chart just for self-administering patients is not necessarily going to be a reasonable alternative. A way around this is to use medication cards designed for self-administration *alongside* the prescription chart. The record of administration can then be carried out informally with the nurse discussing medication with an individual patient on an informal basis to establish that the patient is comfortable with his or her prescription. The nurse can then tick the prescription chart for that day.

## PROCEDURES FOR THE SELF-ADMINISTRATION PROGRAMME

The introduction of any new service requires the design of procedures so that all the people involved in the service know exactly what is happening. The procedures will aid smooth induction for new staff joining the team and provide direction if problems should arise. It is important to contact all the people involved in the self-administration programme before designing the procedures as there will be relevant input required from them. The following list of procedures that should be considered is not exhaustive; rather it concentrates on those procedures where pharmacy input is essential if they are to be universally accepted.

### 1.  Patient assessment

The type of patient normally treated on the ward will govern whether a formal assessment is required to allow participation in a self-administration programme. On specialist wards it may be the policy that all patients admitted will automatically self-administer, and the patients can be informed of this prior to admission. Those wards which care for elderly patients, people with rheumatoid arthritis or short stay surgical patients are ideal for this approach. If a general medical ward is used, however, then not all patients admitted will be suitable for self-administration (it would be inappropriate for acutely ill or confused patients, for example). In this situation an assessment of patients' ability to self-administer their medication would be desirable, and assessment should be continued throughout their stay.

The pharmacist's assessment must include a record of the patient's ability to do the following:

- Open child resistant closures.
  (If the patient is unable to open the bottle with a child resistant closure on, a normal cap can easily be fitted.)
- Read the label.
  (With the computer-generated labels that are now used some people experience great difficulty deciphering the print. Increasing the print size or using a word processor to generate labels with larger print can be used to overcome this. Special Braille labels are available for blind people.)
- Understand the label.
  (The simple concise directions printed on the label can be interpreted in different ways by different people. For example, 'ONE to be taken

SIX hourly' could be interpreted as six hourly during the working day so only three doses are actually taken (Cowderoy and Coker, 1987), rather than four over a 24 hour period. The direction 'Before food' means that medication is taken on an empty stomach *at least 30 minutes* before food – not, as it could be interpreted, immediately before a meal.)

If the patient has a problem understanding the label then the pharmacist can make sure that the English used on the label is understood by the patient.

## 2. Storage of medication

Storage of the medication in the self-administration programme is a vital component and, as such, often causes the most debate and can be the stumbling block to introducing a programme. Consultation between the medical, pharmacy and nursing staff at a senior level can lead to the agreement of an established system that satisfies all parties. This can then provide the template for a written procedure. Some of the aspects that will need to be covered include the responsibility for the storage of medication on the ward, which will undoubtedly fall to the sister in charge in liaison with the chief pharmacist for the hospital. The procedure must include safeguards to minimise the risk of abuse of the self-administration programme.

Where patients store their medication in their own locker (without a lock) then safeguards would include suspending self-administration if a patient on the ward is wandering and rifling through other patients' lockers. Where the programme incorporates locked storage, the persons holding the key and spare must be identified, and there should be a policy covering what must be done if one of the keys is misplaced. (Is the lock changed, for example?)

To make the introduction of the self-administration programme easier then a well designed procedure on the storage of medication will go a long way to reducing some of the concern and objections that will be raised. It may be decided to introduce medication to patients in stages with them finally looking after their own medication; the storage of medication in the different stages would have to be detailed.

## 3. Patient counselling

The patient counselling interview has already been well covered in terms of the information to be provided. There should still be a procedure to identify how the interview should take place. The exact role of each of the health care professionals involved needs to be listed. It is important to identify how 'problem patients' need to be approached – for example, if a patient is having a recurrent problem with his or her medication then the nurse must get the pharmacist involved.

The procedure should also cover an overview of the type of information that will be provided to the patient and whether written information is to be used. If information sheets are available, are they for direct issue to the patient or are they for the nursing staff when counselling the patient? This may be applicable where a member of the medical staff expresses concern on the type of information that is passed on to his or her patients. Incorporation of these areas will identify what topics must not be covered during the counselling interview with these patients. Further negotiation and subsequent alteration of the procedure may well be required as the self-administration programme develops.

## 4.   The dispensing process in self-administration

Procedures in the pharmacy must be designed to cover the dispensing of self-administration prescriptions. The areas to be addressed by the protocol will include:

- Duration of therapy to be dispensed.
- Identification of prescriptions that are required for patients self-administering.

The amount of medication dispensed can help to reduce the workload in the pharmacy, because by issuing an appropriate supply which will also cover the patient's discharge medication, time will be saved. For patients likely to remain in hospital for a week, 14 days' supply would be sensible. A smaller supply could be calculated for shorter stay patients.

Attaching a special sticker to a prescription will indicate that the prescription belongs to a patient who is self-administering his or her drugs. This is important because the dispensary staff can then make sure that the bottles contain the appropriate quantity and that the labelling includes the directions on how to take the medication.

### THE MAJOR ROLE OF THE PHARMACIST IN SELF-ADMINISTRATION PROGRAMMES

Self-administration requires a team approach if it is to be introduced and accepted at the ward level. The different health care professionals will have different roles to play to ensure the success of the programme. There are particular components of self-administration that require pharmaceutical advice and input and these topics will be covered in the following sections.

### Storage of medication

The Duthie Report (1988) states that storage of medication in the hospital is under the advice of a senior pharmacist in liaison with the senior nurse on the ward, and where self-medication exists the use of lockable, immovable

lockers is recommended where possible. Thus, before any self-administration scheme can go ahead, the pharmacy, in liaison with senior nursing
staff, needs to establish exactly how the medication will be stored.

Among the methods that have been employed is storage of the medication
in the normal drug trolley. In this situation the patients come and request
the trolley to be opened or, alternatively, there is a time (like a drug round)
when the trolley is open and patients request their medication (Corrigan,
1989). This situation is not without its problems as there is still an external
stimulus reminding patients that their medication is due. One way around
this would be to use a special trolley with patients' medication in a labelled
drawer (Owen et al., 1987; Walker and Martin, 1987). Patients can then
come and request their medication at the appropriate times without the
external stimulus although this can be very time-consuming for the nursing
staff. Providing patients with keys to their own drawer in the trolley would
remove this element with patients having access to their medication outside
normal drug round times and without chasing nurses around the ward for
the keys.

It may be possible to fix a lock to patients' lockers and they can keep their
medication by their bedside. This provides easier access for patients and a
greater sense of control for them without requiring them to be mobile.
However there may be problems with the use of lockable systems on
account of the manual dexterity of those selected for the self-administration
programme. Patients with rheumatoid arthritis or Parkinson's disease, and
some other elderly patients may not be able to open the locker. Also there
is the problem of the key being lost or misplaced, with the decision being
made as to whether a new lock is required or whether it is appropriate to
have a replacement key only.

Another approach would be for patients to keep their medication in their
bedside locker but without a lock on it. In such a case, the patients store
their own medication out of sight and take responsibility for it while they
are in hospital. They have access to their medication when they want it
without the stimulus of formal drug rounds or the attentions and reminders
of the nursing staff. I would suggest that storage of medication in this
manner fulfils the whole ideal of self-administration. This is the method of
storage that we have chosen to use in Oxford.

## Medication history

The medication history interview usually receives a few lines in the doctor's
admission notes as it is a small part of the clerking process and is quite
often neglected. At best the patient's current medication will be recorded
although this can be difficult to ascertain, particularly if there is no referral
letter available. The presence of a referral letter does not guarantee that
drug details will be included. One study of GP referral letters found that up
to 36% contained no details about the patients' medication (Holmes et al.,

1984). There are reports of in-patient medication records being just as bad (Feely *et al.*, 1984).

Pharmacists have been involved in medication history taking (Titcomb, 1989) and there are studies that suggest pharmacists to be superior to physicians in this field (Badowski *et al.*, 1984; Wilson and Kabet, 1971). The information that should be obtained from a drug history interview should include:

- The number of prescribed drugs taken immediately prior to admission.
- The number of self-prescribed drugs taken prior to admission.
- A complete drug history for the above drugs (e.g. how long they have been taken, frequency of dose, any problems/side-effects) and for other medication taken in the past.
- Identification of medicines.
- Any allergies to other drugs or food.
- Compliance with prescribed medication.
- Use of other people's medication.

This list is not exhaustive but provides an insight to the topics that need to be covered in a full drug history-taking exercise (Ranelli *et al.*, 1989). The other advantage to be gained with the pharmacist taking the drug history interview is their knowledge of the appearance and description of the drugs. The process of establishing the identity of an agent taken in the past involves quite a bit of detective work. The outcome of the medication history interview should provide a complete list of the drugs a patient has consumed in either the past or the present, side-effects or adverse events related to them and whether they were prescribed or self-purchased.

The programme provides the ideal opportunity for the pharmacist to introduce a medication history-taking service which will become a vital component of self-administration.

**Patient counselling**

The counselling interview provides information to the patient on the correct use of his or her medication. It is vital in establishing the confidence of patients in their prescription which helps to ensure that they take their medication as intended. Doctors, pharmacists and nurses all give information to patients about their medication in varying amounts as discussed earlier. Self-administration allows all the health care professionals to see one patient at the same time allowing the continuity of information. Therefore when only one of these professionals visits the patient at a later date the information is reinforced rather than contradicted.

It is very important to decide what information should be imparted to the patient to ensure their understanding and subsequent compliance with their prescribed regimen. The following list is a guide to the main areas that should be covered:

1.   The name and description of the medicine
Ensure the name on the bottle is used (e.g. ibuprofen could be Brufen).
This will often be the generic drug name in the hospital setting (ibuprofen
in the example above), but is likely to be the trade name in the community
(Brufen in the example above).

2.   The purpose of the medication
This area needs to be covered carefully although in the hospital environment the pharmacist and nurse will know whether a patient is aware of his
or her diagnosis. When patients are unaware of their diagnosis then it is
the role of the doctor to initially discuss this with them. The nurse
and phamacist would undermine the doctor/patient relationship if they
did this at the initial stage. The discussion may include whether the
medication will treat the disease or just alleviate the symptoms of the
disease. Information on how the patient can tell whether the medication
is working may be appropriate.

3.   How often should the medication be taken?
The administration frequency should be adapted to the patient's lifestyle
wherever possible. It is important to make sure that the patient has
interpreted the directions correctly and that dosage intervals are evenly
spaced throughout the day.

4.   How should the medication be taken?
This will include any special instructions such as when the medication
should be taken in relation to food, whether it needs to be swallowed
whole, whether it may cause drowsiness etc.

5.   For how long must the medication be taken?
The answer to this will vary depending upon the medication prescribed
and the condition being treated. Antibiotics are generally taken for a
short course (there are exceptions), whereas some replacement therapies
will be lifelong. It would be prudent at this stage to advise the patient not
to stop taking the medication unless directed to do so by their doctor.

6.   What side-effects may arise?
When discussing the side-effects it is important to select only those that
are common or dangerous. A quick read of the British National Formulary
quite rightly produces an extensive list of side-effects, some of which are
extremely rare. It requires expertise and specialist knowledge to identify
those which the patient must be warned about. This falls within the role
of the pharmacist or the doctor. It is also important to inform the patient
how to react if a particular side-effect develops. The more serious side-
effects require that the patient seeks medical advice immediately, whereas
the less severe can be communicated either at the patient's next doctor's
appointment or at an appointment that has been brought forward.

7.  Effects of medication on driving and work
Some medication can impair individuals' mental performance and reaction times, which can cause serious problems if they are driving or operating machinery. Patients *must* be informed of this so that they are aware if there is a potential problem.

8.  What to do if a dose is missed
The advice offered will depend on the type of medication and how frequently it is taken. Medication taken three to four times a day if remembered two to three hours later could be taken, with the remaining dosage times for that day delayed accordingly. Medication that is taken only once a day if remembered later in the day could be taken at that later time. The important message must be to make sure that the patient does not take twice the dose to make up at the next administration time.

9.  Interactions with alcohol or concurrent medication
'Can I drink while taking this medicine?' This is a common question asked of pharmacists, particularly around the Christmas period. The answer depends on the type of medication that has been prescribed and the patient's medical problems. For some medication then the odd drink will not be harmful, but the effects of other medication can be markedly enhanced when mixed with even small quantities of alcohol. The advice offered must be tailored to each individual patient. Patients who are receiving a drug that undergoes a number of clinically significant drug interactions should be advised to remind their doctor when he or she prescribes for them that they are taking this particular drug. Just as importantly, drugs that can be purchased 'over the counter' that interact with other medications they are taking must be brought to their attention. It is not unknown for patients on co-proxamol (dextropropoxyphene/paracetamol) to purchase and administer further paracetamol. Patients on warfarin should be counselled very strongly against purchasing aspirin or any preparation containing aspirin because it potentiates anticoagulant effect.

10.  Storage and disposal of medication
Medication taken at the prescribed dose is effective but in overdose can be lethal. Children who get their hands on their parents' or grandparents' medication will be taking an overdose if they consume it. To avoid this, it is vital that patients are counselled to keep their medication out of reach of children. They should also be advised to take any excess medication either to their local pharmacy or to their local hospital pharmacy department.

11.  Don't share medication
Patients should always be advised that, although their medication is working for them, it would not necessarily benefit a friend, neighbour or relative. In fact the effect could be far from beneficial, so they must not share out their medication.

During the patient counselling interview every effort must be made to put the patient at ease. If the counselling interview fails in any way then the whole scheme of the self-administration will fail.

We have discussed the verbal side of the counselling interview and now the provision of written information in this setting needs to be considered. The number of patient information leaflets supplied with dispensed medication is on the increase, but this information leaflet may be too complex for inclusion in the initial interview. It may be more appropriate to leave it with the patient to be read at leisure. The patient can then discuss any queries that he or she may have at a later date. However, in the interview, a simplification of the patient information leaflet may be introduced at this stage to back up the verbal information given. One method is to use a patient medication card which has all the drugs written on it along with directions for taking them, special instructions, side-effects and how long they should be taken for (see Chapter 4). This is filled in during the counselling interview providing a quick reference for the patient and reinforcing what was said.

An alternative is to use locally produced information leaflets but these are more efficiently used where the self-administration is on a specialist ward where a small finite number of drugs are used. The design of such leaflets is a time-consuming business with their use probably needing approval from the multidisciplinary team and the drugs and therapeutics committee.

The next question is, 'Who should counsel patients on the use of their medication?' One of the traditional roles of the pharmacist, both in the hospital and in the community, is to advise patients on their medication. The pharmacist at the bedside is a more common sight in hospitals as they take on a more clinical role as advocated in the Duthie Report (1988) and by the Department of Health (1988), bringing their expertise and knowledge on drug therapy to the patient. The pharmacist has a major role to play in the counselling of patients in the self-administration scheme and this, in turn, contributes to improved job satisfaction for the pharmacist. The pharmacist, however, is not going to be in contact with the patient as often as the nurse who has a major role both in answering patients' questions and in reinforcing the information imparted by the pharmacist at the first counselling interview. The pharmacist will review the patient on a referral basis for a particular problem and certainly prior to discharge.

The self-administration programme brings together three health care professionals: the doctor to inform the patient of his or her condition, the pharmacist to counsel the patient on his or her medication and the nurse to reinforce the information given by the other two and address questions that the patient may raise. If a medication card is available, this can be used in the community to further reinforce the information process started in the hospital, preserving the concordance of the information. The team of health care professionals involved in the self-administration programme also involves our colleagues in the community, all of whom are vital to the success of the scheme.

Introduction of self-administration programmes into the hospital setting is a vital part of patient care. Improving their education and understanding of their disease and why they are taking the medication will increase the likelihood that they fulfil their prescription. The self-administration programme will improve the quality of care given to the patient and, as such, its introduction into everyday practice should be seriously considered.

# 8

# Self-medication: issues of accountability

## INTRODUCTION

> Accountability is an integral part of professional practice, since, in the course of that practice, the practitioner has to make judgements in a wide variety of circumstances and be answerable for those judgements.
>
> (Exercising Accountability – UKCC, 1989)

Accountability has become an increasingly significant word in nursing. This significance stems from several distinct yet related factors. Firstly, the clinical grading exercise became a process where the degree of responsibility within roles was scrutinised. Secondly, the UKCC Code of Conduct guidelines on accountability were published in 1989 to emphasise and clarify the central nature of accountability to the Code of Professional Conduct (UKCC, 1984). Thirdly, there has been an increasing preoccupation by nurses to construct philosophies of practice that attempt to define the nature of nursing practice. Central to such philosophies is the concept of individualised care that focuses the organisation of care around meeting individual patients' needs as opposed to the previous dominant nursing norm of routinisation with its orientation for managing a workload, and fourthly, the emergence of primary nursing that focuses the responsibility for individual patient care on one nurse with subsequent accountability, this sweeps away a culture of diffuse accountability. This focus on the responsibility of individual practitioners for the care of individual patients is, of course, the language of primary nursing. For example, Manthey (1980: p. 31) states that the allocation and acceptance of individual responsibility (nurse) for decision making to one individual (patient) is one of four key characteristics of a primary nursing system for organising care.

Each of these four factors can be seen as an effort by the nursing profession to enhance its professional identity. For example, the recent 'Strategy for Nursing' (Department of Health Nursing Division, 1989) encourages primary nursing as the way forward for organising nursing based on the need 'for each patient admitted to hospital to be assigned to the care of named nurses as an important contribution to securing individualised and sensitive care'. (p. 12)

The focus on individualised care is central to attempts by nurses to clearly define nursing and to delineate the role of nursing from that of medicine, by emphasising the dichotomy of cure-care and focusing on health rather than disease. The movement to define nursing and emphasise its distinct role from medicine clearly is an attempt to enhance a legitimate claim for autonomy in practice. This should enable nursing to emerge from a long-standing subordinate relationship with medicine.

The UKCC Code of Professional Conduct (1984) and the subsequent guidelines that have been published are an attempt to impose ethical norms on nursing practice in order to regulate the activity of nursing. This activity can be viewed as a response to fulfilling an obligation to society in return for professional status. Again the Strategy for Nursing emphasises that the key to the future development of practice throughout the nursing profession is, 'the recognition of every practitioner's professional accountability and full responsibility for individual patients in every health setting' (UKCC, 1984: p. 12).

In my experience nurses view accountability with generally negative connotations of being held to account for work where warts are exposed and punished. Perhaps nurses generally feel this way because good work has always been taken for granted in nursing and senior nurses have only given junior nurses feedback about poor work.

Research at Burford Nursing Development Unit that focuses on the experiences of nurses becoming primary nurses has demonstrated the phenomenon of 'feeling exposed' as a primary nurse. A nurse commented: 'At — ward, you could just merge into the background, but here . . . there is nowhere to hide'. As a primary nurse she felt exposed. She recognised how accountable she was for her work and how stressful this was for her (Johns, 1991: p. 20).

Perhaps the fear nurses seem to have of being held to account results from a culture in nursing where nursing has constructed a social system that implicitly protects nurses from anxiety associated with their work. Menzies-Lyth (1988) has described the processes whereby responsibility for work becomes diffused within the nursing team and accountability is pushed upwards into the next tier of the hierarchical pyramid and blame passed downwards. Menzies-Lyth also comments on how responsibility for decision making is minimised through a process of constant checks and counterchecks, and how work is routinised around tasks that limit the need to make decisions about care. Nurses were delegated tasks which they were expected to complete effectively. Nursing did not have to think about the nature of nursing to any large extent in that it was, and to a large extent is still, dominated by medical practice. In this respect, teaching patients to take their medication safely prior to discharge was not prescribed by doctors, and nurses dispensed with any responsibility for teaching by thrusting a bag of tablets into the hand of the outgoing patient or relative as they left the ward. Even worse, the patient or relative was asked to collect the medication at the pharmacy on the way out. Pharmacists relinquished any responsibility for teaching patients how to take their medication safely by writing on the label the doctor's instructions to 'Take as directed by the doctor'.

At Burford, practitioners are encouraged to view being held to account as a positive experience, as an opportunity to demonstrate that they are effective practitioners, to celebrate their success. This view is based on the belief that if we are good at something then we should be recognised for that thing. If we could do better, then let us also recognise that and do something about improving our effectiveness. If nursing is primarily for the benefit of patients or clients and their families, then nurses must accept responsibility for ensuring their care is effective and this means being accountable for their actions.

Perhaps the word accountability is the wrong word to focus on in this discussion. A better word might be responsibility.

The reader may have some confusion about the difference between responsibility and accountability. This is an important difference to clarify because the words are often used interchangeably. Bergman (1981) offers a useful explanation (see Figure 8.1).

Bergman's explanation is a useful framework because it emphasises that in accepting responsibility for work, the responsible nurse matches her knowledge, skills, and attitudes against what is required to carry out the work effectively.

Taking self-medication therapy as an example – what knowledge, skills and attitudes are necessary for this work? The answer to this question will largely be found within the text of this book. Yet it is a crucial question that nurses who choose to use self-medication therapy must answer.

Depending on how nursing practice is organised, nurses may be either collectively or individually accountable to patients for the outcomes of

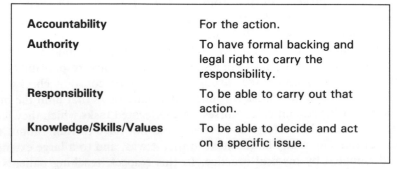

| Accountability | For the action. |
| --- | --- |
| Authority | To have formal backing and legal right to carry the responsibility. |
| Responsibility | To be able to carry out that action. |
| Knowledge/Skills/Values | To be able to decide and act on a specific issue. |

**Figure 8.1**  Accountability in nursing (from Bergman, 1981)

self-medication therapy. Where nurses work in teams or are allocated patients, they will need to clarify amongst themselves who is responsible for planning the self-medication therapy programme with the patient, and to clarify the role of other nurses in carrying out and evaluating this plan of action.

My personal belief is that self-medication therapy is part of a total therapeutic approach to working with a patient. Hence I believe it is important that the patient has the opportunity to maintain continuity of working with one nurse.

Nurses are also accountable to themselves for working to the best of their ability (Styles, 1985). This concept implies that individual nurses are committed to continually improve their ability and actions for the benefit of the patient. For example, the knowledge base for self-medication therapy involves a large number of research studies. The skills involved in counselling a patient and/or relative involve applying this knowledge using counselling and teaching skills.

Deciding to use self-medication therapy on a nursing unit should not be an ad hoc affair. It needs careful consideration and interprofessional agreement and planning and to be recognised as both an acceptable and desirable practice. In this respect, the practice becomes a goal of the organisation. At Burford, the primary nurses are expected to consider the use of self-medication therapy with every patient.

The nature of professional accountability is defined within the UKCC Code of Conduct (2nd edition, 1974) embraced within the clause:

> Each registered nurse, midwife and health visitor is accountable for his or her practice, and, in the exercise of professional accountability shall . . .

The Code continues with 14 clauses that identify aspects of practice where the nurse is accountable for her actions. Of these 14 areas, the following four clauses are discussed in this chapter in relation to accountability and the therapy of self-medication.

**Clause number**

1.  Act always in such a way as to promote and safeguard the well-being and interests of patients/clients.

2.  Ensure that no action or omission on his/her part or within his/her sphere of influence is detrimental to the condition or safety of patients/clients.

5.  Work in a collaborative and co-operative manner with other health care professionals and recognise their particular contributions within the health care team.

10. Have regard to the environment of care and its physical, psychological and social effects on patients/clients, and also to the adequacy of resources, and make known to appropriate persons or authorities any circumstances which could place patients or clients in jeopardy or which militate against safe standards of care.

CLAUSE 1

**Act always in such a way as to promote and safeguard the well-being and interests of patients/clients.**

As part of any debate about the responsibility of nursing to promote self-medication therapy, a key issue is how the nursing unit perceives and defines its role in relation to acting in the best interests of patients or clients.

Without a clear understanding of nursing's role, it becomes difficult to be either responsible for work or accountable for outcomes. Nursing becomes what is prescribed by others, for example the medical profession, or whatever needs to be done or is left over by others.

Taking my own practice as an example, the philosophy for practice at Burford recognises that one role of the hospital is to help maintain people in their own homes. Ten per cent of elderly patients experience adverse drug reactions severe enough to cause them to be admitted to elderly care units (Shulman, 1989). Hospitalisation provides an ideal opportunity for the practitioner both to review the drug regimen and to assess the clients' abilities to administer their medication safely.

Burford's philosophy for practice identifies the hospital's key role in working with patients to help them manage and control their own health experiences. This is a key function in respite care, rehabilitation and even terminal care. It would seem absurd to dispense drugs to a person in hospital who is capable of taking his or her own medication. Equally, if the hospital claims to rehabilitate patients then this must surely involve helping them to manage and control their medications as part of their total care.

The emergence of nursing philosophies and nursing models redefines nursing work. From this redefinition the practice of self-medication therapy may emerge as significant from different philosophical ideals. For example, one ideal is recognising the responsibility to prepare people to manage their health at home safely following discharge. It is well known that readmission to hospital is often due to non-compliance or mismanagement of their drug regimen. Not only is this a health risk to the individuals concerned but represents a financial and organisational strain on the health service.

Self-care is a powerful ideal within the beliefs that underpin various models of nursing, the most obvious example being Orem (1980). From this perspective, the return to health is matched by an increasing return to self-care and increasing independence from nursing assistance. The logic of this perspective is that patients would at the appropriate time regain self-care of their medications. Similarly, models of nursing that espouse an activity of living perspective, for example the Roper, Logan and Tierney model (1980), would naturally use a similar logic whereby taking medication is identified as a preventing activity within the relevant activity of living.

'Promoting well-being' is a clear indication of nursing's role to promote health education. This is a clear mandate for nurses to teach people to understand and manage their medication. At least from Burford's perspective, the arguments for nursing to help patients self-medicate are undeniable to the extent that failure to help patients with this aspect of care could be viewed as negligent. Thorne and Robinson (1988) have recognised that patient satisfaction with care is related to having competence recognised by health care workers. Recognising competence to self-medicate whilst in hospital may therefore increase trust between patients and nursing staff thus increasing patient satisfaction with care.

The Government's guidelines on discharge (Department of Health, 1989) emphasise a clear responsibility for the management of hospitals to ensure that patients are discharged to a safe environment of care. An environment that is not conducive to the patient being able to self-medicate safely could again be viewed as unsafe and hence discharging a patient under these circumstances may be considered as negligent. However, the guidelines make a distinction between medical care and all other care, and this raises the question of whose responsibility it is to ensure that patients can take their medication safely, and to minimise the possibility of non-compliance.

Clearly, the responsibility for compliance rests with the patient. Nurses cannot be held to account if patients choose not to comply with their medication therapy. The nurse's responsibility is to minimise the risk of non-compliance occurring. No matter what actions nurses take to minimise the risk of non-compliance, some patients will fail to comply with their prescribed drug regimen.

The UKCC (1986) Guide to Administration of Medicines outlines the doctor's role as 'obtaining a patient's consent based on an understanding of the treatment and issuing a prescription . . .'. This guide identifies the role of the nurse as 'assessing and promoting the patient's knowledge and understanding regarding his/her medication, and reinforcing safety; this is essential before the patient can progress to independence' (UKCC, 1986: p. 10).

This clause offers nursing a clear mandate to promote self-medication therapy with patients. However, it cannot be assumed that there is a set way of 'doing self-medication'. My experience of working with self-medication therapy suggests that different patients have different needs that demand both a comprehensive and an individual approach to self-medication based on knowledge. It is also clearly in the patient's best interests to have the knowledge to take his or her medication safely. This applies both in hospitals and in the community. The guide comments that 'the visiting practitioner does have a responsibility to assist the patient's understanding and help ensure safe administration and to ensure the patient understands the treatment, the need to complete the prescribed course and has consented to receiving it . . .'.

### CLAUSE 2

**Ensure that no action or omission on his/her part or within his/her sphere of influence is detrimental to the condition or safety of patients/clients.**

The focus of this clause in relation to self-medication therapy is on safety. This focus is illustrated with two case studies.

### Mrs Brock

Mrs Brock was admitted to Burford with a fractured arm. She had a very poor memory and she compensated for this by writing important information in her diary. Following discharge she was moving to Scotland to be cared for, therefore her support at home was no longer relevant. Mrs Brock's primary nurse had omitted to work with her to help her safely self-medicate in preparation for discharge. This omission was picked up the day before departure and a calendar was talked through with her. A calendar is a visual reminder for the patient on which medication to take at what times. The calendar used at Burford also gives information on common side-effects, reasons for prescription, and particular precautions, together with standard notes on managing and storing drugs. Fortunately Mrs Brock was used to writing things down, so this form of *aide-memoire* was useful. She demonstrated that she was able to open her bottles satisfactorily. In this instance it was fortunate that the omission to self-medicate did not extend Mrs Brock's stay in hospital.

### Charlotte

Charlotte lived with her husband at home and he was generally dependent on her. She had been prescribed a range of tablets while she was in hospital. Again the primary nurse failed to implement self-medication therapy in good time. It was noticed the day before discharge, when she was given her tablets to self-medicate, that she was unable to get into the blister packs. The packaging was changed and she then demonstrated a failure to get into child-proof bottles. Her poor eyesight necessitated large clear labels for the bottles.

### Commentary

Without a programme of self-medication, these two ladies' particular needs with regard to managing to take their medication successfully would probably not have been identified and certainly would not have been met.

To fulfil the requirements of both the UKCC Code of Conduct and the guidelines on Administration of Medicines, it was the nurse's responsibility to help prepare both of these ladies to take their medication safely following discharge.

In the unlikely event of one of these ladies making a complaint against the hospital, to the effect that she could not take her medication after returning home because she found it impossible to open child-proof bottles, who would be responsible for such poor preparation for discharge? At Burford, the responsibility for this omission of action rests with the primary nurse. If, however, the patient did not take her prescribed tablets because she did not know what they were for, the responsibility is less clear. Presumably, when prescribing the medication, the doctor will have explained the reasons for the choice of this particular drug to the patient. In times of illness, however, patients may not be able to understand, or may easily forget due to anxiety. It would seem imperative that patients do understand the nature of their drug regime in order to make decisions about compliance – within Becker's (1974) health belief model. Therefore, failure to check and reinforce this knowledge would be an act of omission that could jeopardise the patient's well-being and be detrimental to the patient's safety.

### Safety

The nurse's role in safety is implicitly related to knowledge. With regard to self-medication therapy this knowledge includes:

- Knowledge of the drug, and reasons for giving it to the patient.
- Knowledge of dosages and times to be given.
- Knowledge of side-effects and contraindications.
- Knowledge of how to minimise these.
- Knowledge of Health Authority policy/guidelines.
- Knowledge of professional guidance.
- Knowledge of potential risks – either internal or external – to the safety of the patient.

Examples of different aspects of knowledge are highlighted by Shulman (1989). He comments that 'disclosing side effects is, unfortunately still regarded by some as not being in the best interests of the patient'. If patients can recognise side-effects they can learn to act appropriately and hence reduce any risk of the side-effect or treatment by stopping the drug. Shulman points out that informing patients of side-effects needs careful handling to protect them from undue anxiety. He further comments that 'a frequent problem concerns tablets and capsules that are likely to stick in the oesophagus of elderly patients'. This is just one example of information that patients need to have in order to manage their self-medication safely. Shulman gives us a further example – 'It is dangerous to stop taking some medicines suddenly. Examples are corticosteroids, beta-blockers, and all medicines used to treat hypertension and cardiac complaints'.

From this discussion it can be assumed that the practice of self-medication therapy in itself could threaten the patient's well-being both before and after discharge. Imagine the following scenario: The patient does not take the correct medication, at the correct dosage and at the correct time. This risk can be minimised in various ways. The nurse can use a self-care teaching strategy, for example, a strategy based on self-care that breaks self-medication therapy into stages and moves the patient from dependence on the nurse through teaching, guiding, supporting to self-care. The nurse can check with the patient their ability to succeed safely at each stage before proceeding. This approach to self-care teaching is taken from Ewing's (1983) work with self-care of stoma based on Orem's model of nursing (1980) (cited by Binnie and Roberts, 1984).

Identifying criteria for assessment of risk factors and criteria for counselling patients have been constructed from the research literature and offer nurses a comprehensive and valid checklist for ensuring that no omission occurs. These checklists are currently used in practice at Burford (Figures 8.2 and 8.3).

There is a wide selection of different aids available to assist patients to take their medications safely and nurses need to have access to these. One example is the calendar used at Burford to reduce the risks of patients not taking the correct medication at the correct time.

It can be assumed that, if self-medication is implemented, patients will take their drugs at times most suitable to themselves, as they would do at home. This leads inevitably to a situation where the drug round becomes obsolete, even for patients not self-medicating. Routines in nursing appear an effective way of doing a task: all patients get their drugs at specific times. A danger with loss of this routine is that patients may be overlooked and their drugs are more easily missed (there is some evidence for this at Burford through drug audits).

This risk can be minimised with the adoption of patient-centred allocation (either patient allocation or primary nursing) that focuses care on patients and their needs rather than on the execution of tasks. However, the pervasiveness of nursing-centred practices and routines, in particular, is a culture that is very difficult to change despite changing the way practice is organised around beliefs of individualised care.

The storage of drugs may prove a problem where a risk exists that other patients may have access to them. This is most noticeable at Burford with wandering patients. However, there have been no incidents at Burford where medication kept by patients in a handbag or bedside locker has been interfered with by other patients. This does not remove the potential risk and it is crucial that this risk must be managed.

Two factors need discussing in relation to storage of drugs. Firstly, legislation exists that determines where certain drugs are kept, for example controlled drugs. The Duthie Report (1988) also strongly recommends that drugs are stored in a locked container. Although the report has only the

# Burford Community Hospital
# and Nursing Development Unit

**SELF-MEDICATION STANDARD: Appendix i – criteria for assessment**

| Date | | Initial |
|---|---|---|
| | **A. Usual pattern of drug taking** | |
| | 1. Times drugs usually taken during the day: ................................. | |
| | ................ | |
| | 2. Problems with this: ................................. | |
| | ................ | |
| | 3. Use of self-prescribed drugs: ................................. | |
| | ................ | |
| | 4. Note No. of different drugs taken per day: ................................. | |
| | ................ | |
| | 5. Perceived difficulties in taking drugs: ................................. | |
| | ................ | |
| | 6. Where drugs are stored: ................................. | |
| | ................ | |
| | **B. Dexterity** | |
| | 1. Ability to take prescribed drugs: ................................. | |
| | ................ | |
| | 2. Alternatives: ................................. | |
| | ................ | |
| | **C. Understanding** | |
| | 1. Mental Status Questionnaire: ................................. | |
| | ................ | |
| | 2. Ability to recall specific instructions: ................................. | |
| | ................ | |
| | 3. Ability to convert instructions to action: ................................. | |
| | ................ | |
| | 4. Understanding labels: ................................. | |
| | ................ | |
| | 5. Hearing: ................................. | |
| | ................ | |
| | **D. Sight** | |
| | 1. Ability to read labels: ................................. | |
| | ................ | |
| | **E. Mobility** | |
| | 1. Ability to collect prescriptions from chemist: ................................. | |
| | ................ | |
| | **F. Motivation** | |
| | 1. Assess likelihood of compliance using Becker's Health Belief Model (1974): | |
| | ................ | |
| | **G. Support** | |
| | 1. Identify sources of support for giving medication: ................................. | |
| | ................ | |

**Figure 8.2** Criteria for Assessment (reproduced with kind permission of Burford Community Hospital)

# Burford Community Hospital and Nursing Development Unit

SELF-MEDICATION STANDARD: Appendix iv – criteria for counselling patients

The primary nurse should give the patient and/or Support the following information and seek feedback through recall and observation that it is understood. A copy of the completed guide will reinforce the counselling.
This list has been compiled from Hill (1986) and Wade/Bowling (1986) – see resource file.
McDonald *et al.* (1977) particularly demonstrates the efficacy of counselling patients in respect to self-medication.

| The patient/support knows: | Check list: Patient can answer following questions | | |
|---|---|---|---|
| | Yes/No | Date | Initial |
| 1  What dosage to take | | | |
| 2  To take the drug in a specific manner, e.g. with water, before meals, etc. | | | |
| 3  Specific times to take the drugs | | | |
| 4  For what period of time to take the prescription | | | |
| 5  What to do when the prescription is finished | | | |
| 6  Specific interactions with other drugs | | | |
| 7  How to store the drugs | | | |
| 8  To recognise any expiry date of the drugs | | | |
| 9  The basic reasons the drugs are necessary to take | | | |
| 10  What benefits the patient can expect | | | |
| 11  What to do if no benefit occurs | | | |
| 12  How to recognise unwanted effects of the drugs | | | |
| 13  How to act if they occur<br>– stop taking the drug<br>– report promptly to the doctor | | | |
| 14  Changes of condition that may warrant change of treatment | | | |
| 15  What to do in case of overdosage | | | |
| 16  What might happen if drugs stopped without finishing treatment | | | |
| 17  The need to review use of medication on a regular basis so its effectiveness can be monitored | | | |

**Figure 8.3**  Criteria for Counselling Patients (reproduced with kind permission of Burford Community Hospital)

status of guidelines for good practice it may be prudent to follow these guidelines in the absence of any knowledge to the contrary.

At Burford, we continue to self-medicate despite inadequate storage facilities. The risk is recognised and accepted because of the overriding need to work in this way. Even patients prescribed controlled drugs can self-medicate. The patient asks the nurse to bring the drug from the controlled drugs cupboard and signs the book as necessary. The nurse 'checks' this and signs as the witness. Furthermore the potential risk is assessed and managed by the nurse who is responsible for working with the patient. Because risk is assessed and managed mistakes are less likely to occur. If mistakes do occur, then the nurse would have to demonstrate how she had planned to manage the risk.

Risk is heightened by unhelpful management practices that do not, or will not, understand self-medication. Where nurses feel they are not supported by management, then this lack of support will increase the fear of making mistakes. The implementation of new therapies always involves some degree of risk, yet the therapeutic benefits of self-medication will always offset this risk. Risk is only a problem where it is not recognised and managed effectively.

CLAUSE 5

**Work in a collaborative and co-operative manner with other health care professionals and recognise their particular contributions within the health care team.**

Working with patients to achieve an effective self-medication therapy will depend on establishing collaborative and co-operative relationships with other health workers, most notably doctors and pharmacists. Collaborative and co-operative relationships are dependent on role clarification that is crucial to autonomy and accountability (Singleton and Nail, 1984).

The pharmacist writes instructions on labels for patients concerning dosage, administration, and storing of drugs. As such, should the pharmacist be responsible for teaching and ensuring the patient is able to self-medicate safely prior to discharge? An increasing clinical role of pharmacists is becoming a reality in many hospitals and they may assume that this work should rightly be their responsibility. Yet the process of self-medication is a continual process reinforced and developed each time the patient takes medication. The reality is that the nurse is always with the patient, at least in hospital. In setting up a strategy to implement self-medication therapy, possible conflict of role needs to be negotiated and agreement reached concerning responsibility and the boundaries of accountability.

Pharmacists are experts on side-effects and the responsible nurse should use this expertise. As Shulman (1989) comments, 'it is always helpful to be able to discuss with pharmacists [knowledge of side effects] as they are constantly receiving up-dated information in this area' and, 'if written information is thought to be necessary, consult with a pharmacist and agree a format for a particular drug which will act as a reminder or a memory aid'.

The issue of whether the doctor or nurse is responsible for informing the patient why a particular medication has been prescribed has already been discussed. However, nurses are not primarily responsible for giving patients this information; it is the responsibility of the doctor. This certainty is based on the description of the doctor's prescribing role in the UKCC guidelines on the Administration of Medicines (Clause 2a). Doctors have the overall responsibility for telling a patient what the drug is for. Unfortunately they do not always fulfil this role, for example, if they do not want to tell a patient his diagnosis. With self-medication therapy, it is crucial that patients are informed of the reasons for their medications in order for them to comply. The nurse may insist to the doctor that the patient is told why each drug has been prescribed, assisted by the research that suggests that such information is useful in increasing compliance.

Being assertive with doctors may be difficult for the nurse, however. It may be easier not to ask patients why they are taking their drugs and wait for them to ask. But do nurses fulfil their responsibility to patients in this way? The response to being asked by a patient about his or her medication will usually involve the nurse in determining what knowledge the patient has – by asking, for example, 'What has the doctor told you?' In reality, of course, the nurse makes a judgement on what to tell the patient based on these variables and his or her knowledge of the patient. Professional judgement is defined by the UKCC (1986) as follows:

> Professional judgement in health care is personal judgement based on special knowledge and skill, and always and above all is exercised in the best interests of the patient or client.

Many nurses, including the nurses at Burford, assume this responsibility, yet such autonomy becomes easier with role clarification and dialogue between professionals. The emphasis in the last sentence is between professionals. Any suggestion that nurses are accountable to doctors for their actions is resisted. Henderson (1966) has described nurses working in different modes – independent, interdependent, and dependent upon doctors and other health workers. I see no value in such distinction. Nurses only work interdependently with other health professionals. The nurse is accountable to the patient for working effectively using self-medication, not to the doctor for carrying this out.

### Extended or expanded role?

This point raises the issue as to whether self-medication therapy is an extended or expanded role of the nurse. One argument that has some substance is that the giving of information related to administration of drugs (i.e. reasons for prescription and side-effects) is the responsibility of doctors who take action to minimise the non-compliance of patients with their prescription and safeguard against iatrogenic illness. If this argument is valid, then should doctors have to prescribe self-medication? In this case the task of the nurse in carrying out this role fulfils the criteria of the extended role. Rowden (1987) describes the extended role as one which is *not* covered in basic training for the register.

## The extended role

The extended role is defined within the Department of Health document HC(77)22 (DHSS, 1977). This paper identified the circumstances in which the nurse's role could be extended through delegation by the doctor. The circular states: 'Where delegation occurs, the doctor remains responsible for his patient . . . and the nurse is responsible for carrying out delegated tasks competently'.

Work which has hitherto been carried out by doctors ought therefore to be delegated to nurses only when:

- The nurse has been specifically and adequately trained for the performance of the new task and she agrees to undertake it.
- This training has been recognised as satisfactory by the employing authority.
- The new task has been recognised by the employing authority as a task which may be properly delegated to a nurse.
- The delegating doctor has been assured of the competence of the individual nurse concerned.

Support for this role from the Chief Medical Officer and Chief Nursing Officer in the form of a letter accompanied this circular (Yellowlees and Friend 1977). The letter states:

An important aim of management within the NHS is to enable the right sort of care to be given in the most efficient and effective way. If efficiency and effectiveness can be improved by extension of the nurse's role in particular ways and if the necessary provisos can be met, the merits of such extension should be seriously considered, so long as the ability of the nurse to continue to meet the full nursing needs of the patient is safeguarded.

The last part of this statement is a stark reminder of the problems (due to increased workload) that nurses have on some wards with the giving of IV drugs. Problems may occur if nurses take on this extra work of self-medication into already busy lives where the needs of patients are not already being adequately met. If self-medication is an extended role, how can nurses accept such extra work? What other care would suffer?

Firstly, let us look at whether self-medication fits in with this scenario of the extended role. Nurses learn to administer drugs in their basic training, so the giving of drugs except by IV infusion is part of the nurse's normal role. The only aspect of role extension with self-medication is delegating to the nurse the role of informing patients why the doctor has prescribed the various drugs. I can see no clear way the nurse can assume this role. Clearly, however, the role of the nurse is to ensure that patients take their drugs safely as prescribed. This clearly includes self-medication therapy, for without such therapy how can the nurse ensure that patients can take their medication safely following discharge? As long as patients get their drugs as prescribed, I do not see that the way they are administered is an issue that doctors should concern themselves with.

The expanded role follows from an understanding of the nurse's role and is derived from defining the nature of nursing practice. Hence roles such as teaching and counselling patients to manage their own medication become valid within a philosophy for practice that recognises the nursing role in helping patients towards self-care. The expanded role is synonymous with the notion of autonomy, or in other words exercising freedom to practise within defined roles (Batey and Lewis, 1982). The skills associated with assessment, teaching and counselling are (or at least should be) learned as basic skills. Self-medication merely puts together a package of these various skills determined from the research literature, for example, as has been established at Burford.

The argument as to whether self-medication therapy is an extended or an expanded role may be a spurious argument because it is founded in the belief that nurses agree to undertake delegated work from doctors. This position accepts nurses as being accountable for their actions to doctors which is unacceptable. The only acceptable accountability is for health professionals to work together within defined roles for the benefit of the patient and hence accountability for actions is primarily to the patient. To achieve this all health authorities should have clear policies that allow doctors, nurses and pharmacists to practise with confidence. Mutual trust and respect are essential for the successful implementation of new work such as self-medication therapy. As the UKCC Code of Conduct states:

The delivery of care is often a multi-profession and multi-agency activity which, in order to be effective, must be based on mutual understanding, trust, respect and co-operation.

It is self evident that collaborative and co-operative working is essential if patients and clients are to be provided with the care they need and if it is to be of the quality required. It is worthy to note that this concept of teamwork is evident in many situations in which the care of patients is a shared responsibility. Unfortunately there are exceptions. Experience has demonstrated that such co-operation and collaboration is not always easily achieved if individual members of the team have their own specific and separate objectives or one member of the team seeks to adopt a dominant role to the exclusion of the opinions, knowledge and skill of its other members. In such circumstances it is important to stress that the interests of the patient or client must remain paramount.

Included in the definition of the extended role is the statement:

Acknowledge any limitations of competence and refuse in such cases to accept delegated functions without first having received instruction in regard to those functions and having been assessed as competent.

The nurse has a responsibility to refuse to carry out work unless she has been trained or if she is not sure of her competence, because she is professionally accountable to the patient and in law for her actions. Clearly the practice of self-medication involves a considerable knowledge base by the nurse to be effective in this therapy and such skills cannot be assumed or left to chance. Hence, nurses at Burford are supervised in their practice to ensure effectiveness of self-medication therapy.

**CLAUSE 10**

**Have regard to the environment of care and its physical, psychological and social effects on patients/clients, and also to the adequacy of resources, and make known to appropriate persons or authorities any circumstances which could place patients or clients in jeopardy or which militate against safe standards of care.**

The last point leads into discussing the relationship of self-medication therapy with the availability of resources. The UKCC guidelines on accountability recognise this problem:

It is recognised that, in many situations, there may be a tension between the maintenance of high standards and the availability or use of resources. It is essential, however, that the profession, both through its regulatory body and its individual practitioners, adheres to its desire to enhance standards and to achieve high standards rather than to simply accept minimum standards. Practitioners must seek remedies in those situations where factors in the environment obstruct the achievement of high standards; to start from a compromised position and silently to tolerate poor standards is to act in a matter contrary to the interests of patients or clients, and thus renege on personal professional accountability.

(UKCC, 1989)

The issue of taking on additional tasks to the detriment of other nursing work is not a valid argument. The only valid argument for organising nursing work is around the individual needs of patients that may include either prolonged or minimal self-medication therapy. Where resources are inadequate to meet the total needs of patients, then the UKCC gives the practitioner clear advice as to what action to take. To reject self-medication therapy because of resource implications is a failure of professional role because it clearly puts patients at some risk following discharge. Nursing's responsibility for care cannot stop at the ward entrance. Equally the failure to implement self-medication because pharmacy have not the resources to provide individual patient medications is again clearly unacceptable for similar reasons and must be challenged by the nurse caring for the patient deprived of this opportunity. This scenario further highlights the need for collaborative working between pharmacists and nurses to clarify such resource difficulties. The nurse executes his or her responsibility by making known where resources place patients in physical jeopardy.

### IN CONCLUSION

It is apparent that the nurse has a responsibility to minimise the risk of non-compliance when a patient is discharged from hospital. The most effective method of assessing whether the client is likely to be able to comply must be to allow him or her to self-medicate while in hospital. This will enable the nurse to make a proper assessment of the individual's ability to manage his or her drug regimen safely and will also allow the nurse to resolve any problems before the patient is discharged.

Although nurses remain anxious about personal accountability in relation to self-administration, what must be remembered is that nurses are also accountable for providing the best possible care for their patients. In relation to improving compliance with drug taking, then self-administration therapy is undoubtedly the most appropriate care.

# 9

# Legal aspects of self-medication

---

Whilst self-administration of medicines is the norm in the community it is a practice which is only now being introduced into hospitals. As with anything new the question asked is: 'What if it goes wrong?' The best answer to this is: 'Don't let it go wrong'. This chapter will consider the law of negligence in relation to self-medication.

## WHAT IS NEGLIGENCE?

Well, it is not very difficult to think of common examples of negligence: for example, driving the wrong way down a motorway, letting a child play with a bottle of paracetamol tablets, or leaving a hole in the pavement unguarded and unlit at night.

These examples are so obvious that common sense says they are negligent acts. But where does the law come in? Let us look at the motorway example in further detail. There has been an act, namely that of driving the wrong way. An act is not always required since an omission can lead to negligence, for example failing to warn the driver of your car that the brakes are defective. Whilst driving, there is a duty to take reasonable care to avoid (whether by acts or omissions) causing injury or damage to persons or property which can reasonably be foreseen.

Lord Atkin in the famous case of McAlister (or Donoghue) v Stevenson said:

> The rule that you are to love your neighbour becomes in law, you must not injure your neighbour; and the lawyer's question, who is my neighbour? receives a restricted reply. You must take care to avoid acts or omissions which you can reasonably foresee would be likely to injure your neighbour. Who then in law is my neighbour? The answer seems to be – persons who are so closely and directly affected by my act that I ought reasonably to have them in contemplation as being so affected.

Obviously other drivers on the same carriageway at the same time and same place as our maniac are his neighbours. Similarly patients in hospital are the neighbours of the staff of that hospital.

## Taking care

Lord Atkin said, '. . . you must take care to avoid acts or omissions . . .'.
Well how much care should you take? Or, to put it another way, what is the
standard of care that is expected of you?

The answer of course depends upon who you are. That does not mean the
test is a subjective one. If you are possessed of a special skill such as being
a qualified pharmacist or nurse, then you will be judged by the standard of
an ordinary skilled pharmacist or nurse.

In 1954, Mr J. H. Bolam underwent electro-convulsive therapy at Friern
Hospital. He was not given relaxant drugs nor was he manually restrained
save that he was supported on a mouth gag by a male nurse and male nurses
stood on each side of him. During the course of the therapy, Mr Bolam was
hurt. He ended up with both hips dislocated and fractures on each side of
the pelvis. He brought an action for negligence against the Hospital
Management Committee and the case came before Mr Justice McNair in
1957. In those days, unlike today, such cases were tried before a jury. In his
address to the jury the Judge said:

> . . . I must explain what in law we mean by 'negligence'. In the ordinary
> case which does not involve any special skill, negligence in law means
> this: some failure to do some act which a reasonable man in the circum-
> stances would do, or doing some act which a reasonable man in the
> circumstances would not do; and if that failure or doing of that act
> results in injury, then there is a cause of action. How do you test
> whether this act or failure is negligent? In an ordinary case it is generally
> said, that you judge that by the action of the man in the street. He is
> the ordinary man. In one case it has been said that you judge it by
> the conduct of the man on the top of a Clapham omnibus. He is the
> ordinary man. But where you get a situation which involves the use of
> some special skill or competence, then the test whether there has been
> negligence or not is not the test of the man on the top of a Clapham
> omnibus, because he has not got this special skill. The test is the
> standard of the ordinary skilled man exercising and professing to have
> that special skill. A man need not possess the highest expert skill at
> the risk of being found negligent. It is well established law that it is
> sufficient if he exercises the ordinary skill of an ordinary competent
> man exercising that particular art. I do not think that I quarrel much
> with any of the submissions in law which have been put before you by
> Counsel. Counsel for the plaintiff put it in this way, that in the case of
> a medical man negligence means failure to act in accordance with the
> standards of reasonably competent medical men at the time. That is a
> perfectly accurate statement, as long as it is remembered that there may
> be one or more perfectly proper standards; and if a medical man
> conforms with one of those proper standards then he is not negligent.
> Counsel for the plaintiff was also right, in my judgment, in saying that

a mere personal belief that a particular technique is best is no defence unless that belief is based on reasonable grounds. That again is unexceptionable. But the emphasis which is laid by Counsel for the defendants is on this aspect of negligence. He submitted to you that the real question on which you have to make up your mind on each of the three major points to be considered [author's note: the three points being whether Mr Bolam should have been warned of the risk of injury; whether relaxant drugs should have been used; and whether firmer manual restraint should have been used] is whether the defendants, in acting in the way in which they did, were acting in accordance with a practice of competent respected professional opinion, then it would be wrong for you to hold that negligence was established.

Later he went on to say:

A doctor is not guilty of negligence if he has acted in accordance with a practice accepted as proper by a responsible body of medical men skilled in that particular art . . . a doctor is not negligent, if he is acting in accordance with such a practice, merely because there is a body of opinion that takes a contrary view. At the same time, that does not mean that a medical man can obstinately and pig-headedly carry on with some old technique if it has been proved to be contrary to what the majority of informed medical practitioners believe. Otherwise you might get doctors today saying: 'I don't believe in antiseptics. I am going to continue to do my surgery in the way it was done in the eighteenth century'. That clearly would be wrong.

The 'failure to warn' point is looked at later in this chapter in the context of another case. However, on the other two points evidence was produced to support the use of relaxant drugs or the use of firmer manual control. But counter-evidence was also produced, namely that relaxant drugs could have fatal side-effects and that injury could result from firm restraint.

The Judge made the point that the jury was not entitled to give damages based on sympathy and compassion. He also said: 'you must not look through 1957 spectacles at what happened in 1954'. He also went on to quote the words of Lord Denning in the case of Roe *v* Ministry of Health (2) [1954] 2 All E.R. 131:

But we should be doing a disservice to the community at large if we impose liability on hospitals and doctors for everything that happens to go wrong. Doctors would be led to think more of their own safety than of the good of their patients. Initiative would be stifled and confidence shaken. A proper sense of proportion requires us to have regard to the conditions in which hospitals and doctors have to work. We must insist on due care for the patient at every point, but we must not condemn as negligence that which is only misadventure.

The jury found that the Hospital Management Committee had not been guilty of negligence (Bolam *v* Friern Hospital Committee [1957] 2 All E.R. 118).

We make no apology for quoting at length from the Bolam case because its test of the standard of care has in the words of Lord Lloyd, 'always been treated as being of general application whenever a defendant professes any special skill' (Gold *v* Harringey Health Authority [1987] 2 All E.R. 886). It applies to nurses and pharmacists and as a result it is vital to ensure that any self-medication scheme is set up and conducted in accordance with practice that is accepted as proper by a responsible body of skilled nursing and pharmacy opinion.

So in principle there can be more than one method of administering drugs in hospital and both can be proper. One does not have to be wrong if the other is to be right. Obviously there will be circumstances where self-administration is quite wrong, for example where a patient has known suicidal tendencies.

### INFLUENCES OUT FOR CHANGE

The drug trolley has been on the ward for many years but the expectations of many of those who are visited by it have changed.

The introduction of the National Health Service made medical care freely available to all for the first time. Patients were pleased and grateful to receive treatment. They still are, but nowadays there is a growing propensity for consumers to question the providers of any particular service.

As lawyers we have seen the change in our own profession. Clients ask, 'Why?' And of course they are entitled to an answer. When an understandable answer is not forthcoming, one is tempted to the conclusion that the respondent has an imperfect knowledge of the subject. So too with patients, and it is a trend which will continue, and be fostered by increased health education as well as publicity surrounding defective drugs or treatment.

Given these changing times we consider that it could be most inadvisable not to:

- Explain why specific drugs are being given.
- Explain possible side-effects and what to do about them.
- Give advice about the safe storage of drugs.
- Explain why it is important to complete a full course of medication.
- Assess whether or not the patient will be able to manage ongoing medication once discharged.

It is not unimaginable that over the course of time the drug trolley might become an anachronism for some patients in the same way as being bled is today. There is no doubt that being bled would have passed the Bolam test a few hundred years ago, but today?

When the case of Sidaway *v* Bethlehem Hospital Governors [1985] 1 All E.R. 643 came before the House of Lords, Lord Diplock, one of the Law Lords, said:

> The merit of the Bolam test is that the criterion of the duty of care owed by a doctor to his patient is whether he has acted in accordance with a practice accepted as proper by a body of responsible and skilled medical opinion. There may be a number of different practices which satisfy this criterion at any particular time. These practices are likely to alter with advances in medical knowledge. Experience shows that, to the great benefit of humankind, they have done so, particularly in the recent past. That is why fatal diseases such as smallpox and tuberculosis have, within living memory, become virtually extinct in countries where modern medical care is generally available.

## SELF-ADMINISTRATION

The benefits of self-administration are discussed in detail elsewhere in this book. There is also a chapter devoted to patient assessment, which is a most important area. It is vital that more than just lip service is paid to assessment. Time must be taken to explore with the patient the matters raised by the specimen Patient Assessment Form which appears in this book (see page 26).

Proper assessment has to be something more than the quick glance by the pharmacist in the high street store which presumably establishes that, as well as being an adult, you are not likely to overdose on the 100 paracetamol tablets you have just bought.

In order to achieve proper assessment, care must be taken to ensure that the staff concerned know what is expected of them. Proper routines for training and review must be established, adhered to, and monitored. The same is true when it comes to dealing with the Patient Information Leaflets (see page 41). If there is a standard practice with standard checks then the scope for making errors is reduced. With the Patient Information Leaflet there is no point in just saying, 'Sign here, it is just routine'. A proper explanation must be given.

It is desirable that copies of paperwork concerning self-administration which patients receive are retained, or if standard forms are handed over then a record is kept as to what forms have been given.

There is no reason why a failure to supervise staff may not give rise to negligence. In the case of Wilsher *v* Essex Area Health Authority [1988] 1 All E.R. 871 the Court of Appeal found that the trial judge had been correct when he held that a senior house officer who had inserted a catheter into a vein instead of an artery was not negligent, but that the registrar who was called to inspect what he had done was negligent in not spotting the mistake.

It is possible to envisage such a failure to supervise arising within a self-administration scheme. But there are ways of minimising the risks through good management and teamwork without initiative being stifled. The important point is that, should a particular incident lead to court action, it has to be demonstrated that all reasonable steps were taken to minimise the risk of that occurrence in the first place.

You go to the supermarket and, unbeknown to you, an hour previously another customer dropped a bottle of cooking oil on the floor. Walking into the next aisle you slip and injure yourself. Is the store liable to you? The answer is yes, because:

1.  It owes a duty of care to you its customer (the neighbour principle);
2.  The fact that products may get dropped and spilt is reasonably foreseeable;
3.  A customer looking at shelves is not going to be staring at the floor looking for traces of slippery substances.

So, to avoid this scenario what can the store do? Improve quality controls. This could be done by establishing a regular routine for the floor and the aisles to be inspected for safety hazards.

Your case for compensation would not look so strong if it is established that the oil spill took place five minutes before you slipped, that no one had notified a member of staff of the spill, and that the regular aisle and floor inspection had taken place ten minutes before and was not due in that area for another twenty minutes. However, the supermarket just cannot say, 'We inspect the aisles and floor every 30 minutes'. It has to demonstrate that that procedure was in operation on the day of your accident.

If the facts are altered slightly it might be found that you had yourself been negligent and contributed towards your injury. The oil is spilt, the customer who dropped the bottle notifies a member of staff who puts up warning signs which effectively cone off the danger area. You come along an hour later. You see the signs, but ignore them, and then fall. In these circumstances, it could be argued that both you and the store were negligent: the store for not cleaning up a hazard sooner, bearing in mind that warning signs are not foolproof, and you for disregarding an unambiguous warning. Your contributory negligence could reduce the damages you claim to nil.

The principles operating in the above situation apply just as much to a hospital setting. Just handing forms to patients without adequate explanation is like putting up warning signs in the supermarket but then failing to deal with the hazard to which they relate.

To the question, 'Is it all right to encourage self-administration of drugs in hospital?' the lawyer will reply, 'What do you mean by self-administration?'. Once that question is answered the lawyer will ask, 'Is what you have just described accepted as proper by a responsible body of medical opinion?'

Now this book shows that to work effectively any self-administration scheme needs the co-operation of nursing, medical and pharmacy staff. It should be looked at as an integrated system. Remember responsibility for errors can cross departmental boundaries as was shown in the case of Dwyer v Rodrick and Others (*The Times*, 12th November, 1983). In that case Dr Rodrick diagnosed that Mrs Dwyer was suffering from migraine and prescribed sixty Migril tablets, two to be taken every four hours as necessary. The prescription was clearly wrong yet the chemist who dispensed the drugs did not notice the mistake. Mrs Dwyer took 36 of the tablets in six days. She suffered a number of serious injuries including gangrenous necrosis and loss of part of each toe, and peripheral nerve damage. At the end of the day liability was agreed at being 45% to the doctor and 55% to the chemist.

In her chapter of *Medical Negligence* Barbara Young, the District General Manager of Parkside Health Authority, poses the question, 'Why do patients and relatives claim medical negligence?' She goes on to offer the following answer:

In many cases claims of medical negligence arise because some negligent act has taken place which has resulted in damage to the patient. Legal action can also reflect other circumstances. In some cases, patients or relatives institute legal action simply to achieve an explanation of what has happened, having either failed to achieve an explanation that satisfied them through the complaints procedure or not having taken up this procedure. At times, legal action results from feelings of grief and subsequent guilt at the loss or incapacity of a loved one. Resort to legal action seems to act as some sort of absolution for these feelings. Some patients and relatives have impractically high expectations of medical science and take recourse to law where these expectations are frustrated. In some of these cases, where negligence does not appear to have occurred, sitting the complainant down with the clinical staff concerned and providing as full and frank answers as possible may well resolve the situation. (Young, 1990)

Medical treatment constantly balances risk against benefit, the trick is in keeping the balance. The Courts in this country have recognised this and have adopted the Bolam test as a means of accommodating change. As can be seen from the words of Lords Denning and Diplock, the Courts have not laid down legal principles that encourage 'defensive medicine'.

## IN CONCLUSION

It follows that before setting up and implementing a self-administration scheme, proper consultation should take place with all relevant departments. Thorough research should be undertaken to see how schemes work in other hospitals. It must, of course, be remembered that like should be compared with like, while the use of rose-coloured spectacles should be avoided.

Once a scheme has been implemented, it should be monitored to ensure quality control. Moreover, notice should be taken of developments for the good or the bad, reported by other practitioners.

It takes effort to produce quality and progress has its price. The average car of today is safer and much easier to drive than its counterpart of 50 years ago, but it is necessarily a rather more complicated piece of machinery. So, while self-medication helps patients to manage their medication more effectively, it requires a greater input from the pharmaceutical and nursing staff.

# Conclusions

This book has looked at self-administration from a number of different perspectives: nursing, pharmacy and legal. What is apparent is that, although the perspectives are different, the conclusion that self-administration is beneficial to patients is unanimous because of the following elements:

- It incorporates a teaching programme.
- It returns control of drug taking to the patient, therefore promoting patient comfort and involvement.
- It allows clients to 'practise' taking their drugs under supervision.
- It alerts health care workers to any problems which the patient may experience in adhering to a drug regimen.
- It demonstrates trust – which has obvious psychological benefits for the patient and raises morale.

We hope that this book has demonstrated to you that self-administration is not merely concerned with patients taking their own tablets. Rather, it is about changing your whole philosophy of care. It will not only change the way you administer drugs to patients but will also be a catalyst for developing other areas of your practice. The 'spin-offs' from self-administration (for example, improved job satisfaction for all health care workers) are just as important as the benefits to the patient.

All health care professionals have a responsibility to minimise the risk of patient non-compliance with medication. We hope that we have demonstrated to you that this can be achieved through using a self-administration programme with your clients.

There is no way of ensuring that a programme of self-administration is 100% safe; some potential risk will always remain. Risk is only a problem where it is not recognised and managed effectively. Several of the contributors to this book have discussed methods of minimising these risks, for example, by using a framework, a protocol and written documentation. By taking these precautions you are demonstrating that you have taken all due care.

One of the most important things for you to take away from this book is the importance of a multidisciplinary team approach and ensuring that, as a team, you consistently monitor and evaluate the effectiveness of your programme and make changes whenever necessary.

As you will have realised by now, the authors of this book are very enthusiastic and motivated about self-administration and we hope that some of this enthusiasm has affected you, the reader. We wish you every success.

# References

American Society of Hospital Pharmacists (1976) Statement on Pharmacist-Conducted Patient Counselling. In: Gill S K, Fairbrother M and Cullen A M S (1981) Patient Compliance: Aspects of Pharmacy. *Midwife, Health Visitor and Community Nurse,* **17**(2): 52.

Ascione and Raven (1975) In: Meichenbaum D and Turk D C (1987), *Facilitating Treatment Adherence.* New York: Plenum Press.

Association of the British Pharmaceutical Industry (1987a) Data Sheet Compendium. London: Datapharm Publications.

Association of the British Pharmaceutical Industry (1987b) *Information to Patients on Medicines.* Policy Document, October.

Ausburn L (1981) Patient compliance with medication regimes. *Advances in Behavioural Medicine,* Vol. 1, ed. J L Sheppard. Sydney: Cumberland College.

Badowski S A, Rosenbloom D and Dawson P H (1984) Clinical importance of pharmacist obtained medication histories using a validated questionaire. *American Journal of Hospital Pharmacy,* **41**: 731–2.

Batcy M V and Lewis F M (1982) Clarifying autonomy and accountability in nursing service: Part 1. *The Journal of Nursing Administration,* **12**(9): 13–18.

Baxendale C, Gourlay M and Gibson I (1978) A self-medication retraining programme. *British Medical Journal,* **2**: 1278–9.

Becker H S and Maiman L (1975) Sociobehavioural determinants of compliance with medical care recommendations. *Medical Care,* **1**(18): 10–24.

Becker M (1974) The Health Belief Model and sick role behavior. In: Ozuna J (1981) Compliance with therapeutic regimens. *The American Association of Neurosurgical Nurses.* **13**(1): 2.

Benson S (1985) A self-medication survey of elderly patients in hospital. *Occupational Therapy,* **48**(11): 326–8.

Bergman R (1981) Accountability – definitions and dimensions. *International Nursing Review,* **28**(2): 53–9.

Binnie A and Roberts R (1984) The third step of the nursing process – implementation. *The Open University; A Systematic Approach to Care.* Milton Keynes: The Open University Press.

Bird C (1989) A study of the benefits of a self-medication programme for hospital patients. Unpublished dissertation, University of Southampton.

Bird C (1990) A prescription for self-help. *Nursing Times,* **86**, October: 52–5.

Blackwell B (1973) In: Meichenbaum D and Turk D C (1987) *Facilitating Treatment Adherence.* New York and London: Plenum Press.

127

BMJ (1980) Drug information for patients: Keep it simple. *British Medical Journal,* **280**: 1393.

Bradshaw S (1987) Treating yourself. *Nursing Times,* **83**(6): 40–41.

Bream S (1985) Teaching the elderly about drugs. *Nursing Times,* **81**(29): 32–4.

Cameron N and Gregor F (1987) Chronic illness and compliance. *Journal of Advanced Nursing,* **12**: 671–6.

Cartwright A and Anderson R (1981) General practice revisited. In: Wade B and Bowling A (1986) Appropriate use of drugs by elderly people. *Journal of Advanced Nursing,* **11**: 50.

Cherney *et al.* (1967) In: Graham J M and Suppree D A (1979) Improving drug compliance in general practice. *Journal of the Royal College of General Practitioners,* **29**: 399–404.

Clark-Mahoney J P (1984) Self-medication program improves compliance. *Nursing,* December: 41.

Colcher I S and Boss J W (1972) Penicillin treatment of streptococcal pharyngitis: A comparison of schedules and role of specific counselling. *Journal of the American Medical Association,* **222**: 657–9.

Corrigan M S (1989) Primary pharmacy – a patients' self help service. *Pharmaceutical Journal,* **243**: 458–60.

Coutts L (1979) In: McEwen J, Martini C and Wilkins N (1983) *Participation in Health,* p. 191. London and Canberra: Croom Helm.

Cowderoy M and Coker N (1987) Improving patient compliance (1). *Pharmaceutical Journal,* **239**: 95–6.

Cowderoy M and Coker N (1987) Improving patient compliance (2). *Pharmaceutical Journal,* **239**: 129–31.

Cramer J A, Maltson R H Prevey M L, Scheyer R D, Ouellette V L (1989) How often is medication taken as prescribed: A novel assessment technique. *Journal of the American Medical Association,* **261**: 3273–7.

Department of Health and Social Security (1976) *Discharge of Patients from Hospital.* Health Circular HC(89)5. London: HMSO.

Department of Health (1988) *The Way Forward for Hospital Pharmaceutical Services.* HC(88)54. London: HMSO.

Department of Health (1989) *Discharge of Patients from Hospital.* London: HMSO.

Department of Health Nursing Division (1989) *A Strategy for Nursing – Report of the Steering Committee.* London: HMSO.

DHSS (1977) *The Extended Role of the Clinical Nurse – Legal Implications and Training Requirements.* Health Circular HC(77)22. London: HMSO.

Dodds L (1986) Effects of information leaflets on compliance with antibiotic therapy. *Pharmaceutical Journal,* **236**: 48–50.

Drugs and Therapeutic Bulletin (1981) What should we tell patients about their medicines. *Drugs and Therapeutic Bulletin,* **19**: 73–4.

Dunn R B (1987) Hospital stay has limited effect on later drug regimes. *Geriatric Medicine,* **17**(3): 11–12.

Duthie R B (1988) Department of Health Guidelines for the Safe and Secure Handling of Medicines. London: HMSO.

Edwards M and Pathy J S J (1984) Drug counselling in the elderly and predicting compliance. *The Practitioner,* **228**: 291–300.

Ellis D A, Hopkin J M, Leitch A G and Crofton J (1979) Doctors orders: controlled trial of supplementary written information for patients. *British Medical Journal*, 1: 456

Ettlinger P R A and Freeman G K (1981) General practice compliance study: is it worth being a personal doctor? *British Medical Journal*, 282: 1192–4.

Evans L and Spelman M (1983) The problem of non-compliance with drug therapy. *Drugs*, 26: 63–76.

Ewing G (1983) A study of the postoperative nursing care of stoma patients during appliance change. Unpublished PhD thesis, University of Edinburgh.

Falvo D, Woehlke P and Deichmann J (1980) The relationship of physician behavior to patient compliance. *Patient Counselling and Health Education*, fourth quarter: 185–8.

Feely M, Cooke J and Price D (1987) Low dose phenobarbitone as an indicator of compliance with drug therapy. *British Journal of Clinical Pharmacy*, 24: 77–83.

Feely M, Singleton S and McGibney D (1984) The inadequacies of information on current drug therapy in out-patient records. *Journal of the Royal College of Physicians*, 18: 222.

Feinberg J (1988) The effect of patient–practitioner interaction on compliance. *Patient Education and Counselling*, 11: 171–87.

Gartside G (1986) *Alternative Methods of Pain Relief*. London: Baillière Tindall.

George C F (1987) Telling patients about their medicines. *British Medical Journal*, 294: 1566–7.

George C F, Waters W E and Nicholas J A (1983) Prescription information leaflets: a pilot study in general practice. *British Medical Journal*, 287: 1566.

Gibb S (1985) The yellow one is my water pill. *Nursing Times*, 81(5), February 27th: 29–31.

Gill S K, Fairbrother M and Cullen A M S (1981) Patient compliance: aspects of pharmacy. *Midwife, Health Visitor and Community Nurse*, 17(2): 50, 52, 55.

Graham J M and Suppree D A (1979) Improving drug compliance in general practice. *Journal of the Royal College of General Practitioners*, 29: 399–404.

Hall M (1981) Do I take the yellow one after breakfast? *Nursing Mirror*, 77, October 21st, HV supplement: xiii, xvi–xvii.

Harper D C (1984) Application of Orem's theoretical constructs to self-care medication behaviors in the elderly. *Advances in Nursing Science*, 6(3): 29–46.

Hassall J A (1991) Mutual Benefits. *Nursing Times*, 87(18), May 1st: 49–50.

Hatch A M and Tapley A (1982) A self-administration system for elderly patients at Highbury Hospital. *Nursing Times*, 78(20), October: 1773–4.

Haynes R B, Taylor D W, and Sackett D L (eds) (1979) *Compliance in Health Care*. Baltimore: John Hopkins University Press.

Haynes R B, Wang E and Da Mota Gomes M (1987) A critical review of interventions to improve compliance with prescribed medications. *Patient Education and Counselling*, 10: 155–66.

Henderson V (1966) *The Nature of Nursing*, New York and London: Collier MacMillan.

Hermann F, Herxheimer A and Lional N D W (1978) Package inserts for prescribed medicines: what minimum information do patients need? *British Medical Journal*, 2: 1132–5.

Higbee M, Dukes G and Bosso J (1982) Patient recall of physician's prescription instructions. In: Meichenbaum D and Turk D C (1987) *Facilitating Treatment Adherence*, p. 55. New York and London: Plenum Press.

Higson D L (1991) Patient information leaflets (letter) *Pharmaceutical Journal*, **246**: 466.

Holmes G K T, Crisp P, Upton D R (1984) Letters from general practitioners to hospitals. *British Medical Journal*, **289**: 497.

Hulka B S, Kupper L L and Cassel J C *et al*. (1975) Medication use and misuse. *Journal of Chronic Diseases*, **28**: 7–21.

Hursey K (1985) Teaching self-medication. *Nursing Mirror*, **161**, August: 18.

Isaacs B (1979) Don't trust him – he can't cope! *Nursing Mirror*, October 11th: 24–5.

Johns C C (1991) *Becoming a Primary Nurse*. Burford, Oxon: BNDU Publications.

Kallas J (1984) Establishing a self-administered medication program. *Journal of Nursing Administration*, **14**(11): 38–42.

Keeri Szanto M (1979) Drugs or drums: what relieves post-operative pain? *Pain*, **6**: 217–30.

Kellaway G S M and McCrae E (1979) The effects of counselling on compliance-failure in patient drug therapy. In: Scriven L (1987) Self-medication in a surgical ward. *New Zealand Nursing Journal*, **80**(12): 25–6.

Kendrick R and Bayne J R D (1982) Compliance with prescribed medication by elderly patients. In: Ley P (1988) *Communicating with Patients*, p. 63. London: Croom Helm.

Koltun A and Stone G C (1986) Past and current trends in patient noncompliance research: Focus on diseases, regimens-programs and provider-disciplines. *The Journal of Compliance in Health Care*, **1**(1): 21–31.

Kosnar A (1987) Contracting for care. *American Association of Hospital Nurses*, **35**(11): 493–5.

*Lancet* (1987a) Information for patients about medicines. *Lancet*, **2**: 1077–8.

*Lancet* (1987b) Telling patients about their medicines. *Lancet*, **2**: 1064.

Ley P (1988) *Communicating with Patients*. London: Croom Helm.

Lowen N P and Tejani S S (1991) Manufacturers' patient information leaflets (letter). *Pharmaceutical Journal*, **246**: 497.

Macdonald E T, Macdonald J B and Phoenix M (1977) Improving drug compliance after hospital discharge. *British Medical Journal*, **2**: 618–21.

MacGuire J, Preston J and Pinches D (1987) Two pink and one blue . . . *Nursing Times*, **83**(2), January 14th: 32–3.

Manthey M (1980) *The Practice of Primary Nursing*. Boston, Mass: Blackwell Scientific Publications.

McEwen J, Martini C and Wilkins N (1983) *Participation in Health*. London and Canberra: Croom Helm.

McKercher P L and Rucker T D (1977) Patient knowledge and compliance with medication instructions. *Journal of American Pharmacology Association*, **17**(5): 282.

McMahon T, Clarke C and Baille G (1987) Who provides patients with drug information? *British Medical Journal*, **294**: 355–6.

Meichenbaum D and Turk D C (1987) *Facilitating Treatment Adherence*. New York: Plenum Press.

Menzies-Lyth T (1988) The functioning of social systems as a defence against anxiety. *Containing Anxiety in Institutions – Selected Essays*, pp. 43–85. London: Free Associations Books.

Newcomer D R and Anderson R W (1974) Effectiveness of a combined self-administration and patient teaching programme. In: Gill S K, Fairbrother M and Cullen A M S (1981) Patient compliance: aspects of pharmacy. *Midwife, Health Vistor and Community Nurse,* 17(2): 52.

Nuffield Committee of Enquiry into Pharmacy (1986) *Pharmacy: A Report to the Nuffield Foundation* (Chairman, K Clukas). London: The Nuffield Foundation.

O'Hanrahan M and O'Malley K (1981) Compliance with drug treatment. *British Medical Journal,* 283: 298–300.

Orem D (1980) *Nursing: Concepts of Practice* 2nd ed. New York: McGraw-Hill.

Owen D S, James J W and Howard P (1987) Self medication scheme on an elderly ward. *British Journal of Pharmaceutical Practice,* 9(10): 386–90.

Ozuna J (1981) Compliance with therapeutic regimens: Issues, answers, and research questions. *The American Association of Neurosurgical Nurses,* 13(1): 1–6.

Parkin D N, Henney C R, Quirk J and Crooks J (1976) Deviation from prescribed drug treatment after discharge from hospital. *British Medical Journal,* 2: 686–8.

Potter M (1981) Medication compliance – a factor in the drug wastage problem. *Nursing Times,* 77(5), February: 17–20.

Pullar T, Birtwell A J, Wiles P G, Hay A and Feely M P (1988) Use of a pharmacology indicator to compare compliance with tablets prescribed to be taken once, twice or three times daily. *Clinical Pharmacology and Therapeutics,* 44: 540–5.

Pullar T, Kramer S, Tindall H and Feely M (1989) Time to stop counting the tablets? *Clinical Pharmacology and Therapeutics,* 46: 163–8.

Punton S (1985) Self-medication: Burford Nursing Development Unit. *Nursing Times,* 81(42), October 23rd: 45.

Ranelli P, Bomnie L S and Boh L (1989) Factors affecting outcomes of medication-history interviewing by pharmacy students. *American Journal of Hospital Pharmacy,* 46: 267–81.

Rashid A (1982) Do patients cash prescriptions? *British Medical Journal,* 284: 24–6.

Ridout S, Waters W E and George C F (1986) Knowledge of attitudes to medicines in the Southampton community. *British Journal of Clinical Pharmacology,* 21: 707–12.

Roberts R (1978) Self-medication trial for the elderly. *Nursing Times* 76(23), June 8th: 976–7.

Roper N, Logan W and Tierney A. (1980) *The Elements of Nursing.* Edinburgh: Churchill Livingstone.

Rosenstock I (1966) Why people use health services. In Ozuna J (1981) Compliance with therapeutic regimens. *The American Association of Neutosurgical Nurses,* 13(1): 2.

Ross F M (1989) Doctor, nurse and patient knowledge of prescribed medication in primary care. *Public Health,* 103: 131–7.

Rowden R (1987) The extended role of the nurse. *Nursing,* 14: 516–17.

Sackett D L and Haynes R B (1976) *Compliance with Therapeutic Regimens.* Baltimore and London: Johns Hopkins Press.

Scriven L (1987) Self medication in a surgical ward. *New Zealand Nursing Journal,* 80(12): 25–6.

Shulman J (1989) Informing the patient. *Nursing the Elderly,* 1: 1.

Singleton E K and Nail F C (1984) Role clarification: a pre-requisite to autonomy. *The Journal of Nursing Administration*, **14**(10): 17–31.

Sloan P J M (1984) Survey of patient medication information booklets. *British Medical Journal*, **288**: 915-16.

Stimpson G and Webb B (1975) Going to see the doctor. In: Potter M (1981) Medication compliance. *Nursing Times*, **77**(5): 19.

Stone G C (1979) Patient compliance and the role of the expert. In: Koltun A and Stone G C (1986) Past and current trends in patient noncompliance research. *The Journal of Compliance in Health Care*, **1**(1): 22.

Styles M (1985) Accountable to whom? *International Nursing Review,* **32**(3): 73–5.

Thompson T C and Ellenberg M (1987) A self-medication program in a rehabilitation setting. *Rehabilitation Nursing*, **12**(6): 316–19.

Thorne K and Robinson C A (1988) Health care relationships, the chronic illness perspective. *Research in Nursing and Health*, **11**: 293–300.

Titcomb L C (1989) The pharmacist's role in drug history taking. *British Journal of Pharmaceutical Practice*, **11**(6): 186–91.

Todd B (1981) 27 reasons people don't take their meds. *Registered Nurse*, **44**(3): 54–7.

UKCC (1984) *Code of Professional Conduct for the Nurse, Midwife and Health Visitor*, 2nd ed. London: UKCC.

UKCC (1986) *Administration of Medicines. A Framework to Assist Individual Professional Judgement and the Development of Local Policies and Guidelines*. London: UKCC.

UKCC (1989) *Exercising Accountability. A Framework to Assist Nurses, Midwives and Health Visitors to Consider Ethical Aspects of Professional Practice*. London: UKCC.

Wade B and Bowling A (1986) Appropriate use of drugs by elderly people. *Journal of Advanced Nursing*, **11**: 47–55.

Wade B E and Finlayson J (1983) Drugs and the elderly. *Nursing Mirror*, **156**, May: 17–21.

Walker C A and Martin P C (1987) Self medication for the elderly inpatient. *British Journal of Pharmaceutical Practice*, **9**(2): 47–52.

Walshie J M and Dixon A K (1986) Dangers of non-compliance in Wilson's disease. *Lancet*, **1**: 845–7.

Wandless I, Mucklow J C, Smith A and Prudham D (1979) Compliance with prescribed medicines: A study of elderly patients in the community. *Journal of the Royal College of General Practitioners*, **29**: 391–6.

Wilson R S and Kabet H F (1971) Pharmacists initiated patient drug histories. *American Journal of Hospital Pharmacy*, **28**: 49–53.

Wootton J (1975) In: Potter M, Medication compliance. *Nursing Times*, **77**(5): 19.

Yellowlees H and Friend P M (1977) The extending role of the clinical nurse – Legal implications and training requirements. Letter to Area Medical and Nursing Officers ref. CMO(77)10, CNO(77)9. London: DHSS.

Young B (1990) The Occurrence. In: *Medical Negligence*, ed. Powers M and Harris N. London: Butterworth.

Youngren D E (1981) Improving patient compliance with a self-medication teaching program. *Nursing*, March: 22–3.

Zangari M and Duffy P (1980) Contracting with patients in day-to-day practice. *American Journal of Nursing*, **80**(3), March: 451–5.

# Index

*References in bold are to reproductions of printed forms*